Praise for *Navigating Canada's Health Care*

"I'm impressed with *Navigating Canada's Health Care*. While the subject is heavy, the reading is not: You'll be less bewildered, more informed, and well prepared to meet our health system head on when you read this book. Just don't wait to be sick to do so."—*Toronto Sun*

"A practical, user-friendly and comprehensive resource to help you get more out of our health care system. Province-by-province specifics make this book indispensible."—*Homemakers*

"An eye-opening read for anyone frustrated by wait times or how they've been treated by a health professional. Well-written with interesting anecdotes, useful tips, and plenty of resources for more information."—*The Hamilton Spectator*

"Decter and Grosso's book is not just a typical guide for those wanting to get a leg up when dealing with the current health system, but a 'how-to' agenda to ensure that all Canadians get the care we need and the care we deserve."—*The Globe and Mail*

"*Navigating Canada's Health Care* is a refreshing break from the current public-versus-private debate. It is a guide to how things are rather than a judgment of how the system ought to work."—*The Vancouver Sun*

PENGUIN CANADA

NAVIGATING CANADA'S HEALTH CARE

MICHAEL DECTER is a Harvard-trained economist with three decades of experience in senior public and private sector positions. He has served as Deputy Minister of Health in the Ontario government and as cabinet secretary in Manitoba. He is the founding Chair of the Health Council of Canada, a national organization committed to monitoring progress made by governments to improve health care delivery. He is the author of *Healing Medicare: Managing Health System Change the Canadian Way* and *Four Strong Winds: Understanding the Growing Challenges to Health Care*. Michael is also the CEO of Lawrence Decter Investment Counsel Inc.

FRANCESCA GROSSO has been involved in health policy and health care communications for more than 15 years. She served as a non-partisan Senior Policy Adviser and Director of Policy to Tony Clement, Minister of Health and Long-Term Care for the Province of Ontario. Together with Michael Decter, she worked to establish the Health Council of Canada. Francesca is a partner in the health care strategy firm Grosso McCarthy Inc., where she provides counsel to public- and private-sector clients. She lives with her family in Toronto.

Navigating Canada's Health Care

A User Guide to Getting the Care You Need

MICHAEL DECTER AND FRANCESCA GROSSO

PENGUIN
CANADA

PENGUIN CANADA

Published by the Penguin Group

Penguin Group (Canada), 90 Eglinton Avenue East, Suite 700,
Toronto, Ontario, Canada M4P 2Y3 (a division of Pearson Canada Inc.)

Penguin Group (USA) Inc., 375 Hudson Street, New York,
New York 10014, U.S.A.
Penguin Books Ltd, 80 Strand, London WC2R 0RL, England
Penguin Ireland, 25 St Stephen's Green, Dublin 2, Ireland
(a division of Penguin Books Ltd)
Penguin Group (Australia), 250 Camberwell Road, Camberwell,
Victoria 3124, Australia
(a division of Pearson Australia Group Pty Ltd)
Penguin Books India Pvt Ltd, 11 Community Centre, Panchsheel Park,
New Delhi – 110 017, India
Penguin Group (NZ), 67 Apollo Drive, Rosedale, North Shore 0632,
New Zealand (a division of Pearson New Zealand Ltd)
Penguin Books (South Africa) (Pty) Ltd, 24 Sturdee Avenue, Rosebank,
Johannesburg 2196, South Africa

Penguin Books Ltd, Registered Offices: 80 Strand, London WC2R 0RL, England

Published in Penguin Canada paperback by Penguin Group (Canada),
a division of Pearson Canada Inc., 2006
Published in this edition, 2009

2 3 4 5 6 7 8 9 10 (OPM)

Manufactured in the U.S.A.

Library and Archives Canada Cataloguing in Publication data available upon request to the publisher.

ISBN: 978-0-14-305046-9

For our fathers, Dr. Percy Decter
and Dr. Roberto Grosso.
They dedicated their lives to practising medicine and
to old-school values. In their day, they travelled many
miles, often in extreme winter temperatures, to provide
house calls to the sick. They would also rush to the
hospital at all hours of the night to provide urgent care.
We hope that Percy and Roberto would be pleased
at our modest effort to help empower Canadians
with some basic inside knowledge
on how to get better, faster, safer care.

Contents

Authors' Note

Although this book has been written in the third person, we each authored different chapters according to our knowledge and interest areas. Now and again, we have contributed personal stories to each other's chapters. The constructive collaboration between us helped shape the overall book.

Michael Decter authored the following chapters:

- Getting the System to Help You Stay Healthy
- Boomer Maintenance
- Tips for Managing Chronic Disease
- Coping with Cancer
- Navigating Canadian Health Care—Swiftly
- Navigating Canadian Health Care—Safely
- Be the Squeaky Wheel—How to Complain Successfully

Francesca Grosso authored the following chapters:

- Having a Baby in Canada
- Getting the Best Care for Your Child
- Child Safety in Canada
- Navigating Your Benefits Plans
- Claiming Medical Expenses on Your Tax Return
- Navigating Health Care for Seniors
- Navigating End-of-Life Care

Introduction: Rules for Navigators

Wouldn't it be wonderful if the only time we had to worry about navigating our way through the health care system was when our own health was at stake?

But this is not reality. The fact is that each one of us is called upon to help our loved ones—children, parents, spouses, and friends—when they need to interact with a complex, almost cryptic health care system. And our health care system is becoming even more complex day by day. This complexity has its roots in new treatments, new drugs, and changing coverage rules. And most of us are utterly ill-equipped to provide such direction when it is needed most. For this reason, this user guide to the Canadian health care system takes you on a walk through the stages of life:

- The early years (including pregnancy)
- The middle years
- The senior years

It provides a guide to navigating the system more effectively. It will equip you with information on how things work and what to expect so you can provide greater support for yourself and your loved ones.

The lyric poet John Masefield wrote in "Sea Fever," "All I ask is a tall ship and a star to steer her by." In the modern age of ocean sailing, it is more common to rely on Global Positioning Systems (GPSs) to know precisely where you and your ship are sailing, rather than relying on seeing the stars. In simpler times you could successfully navigate the health system just by having a good family doctor and knowing the location of the nearest hospital. Today that is not enough. Health care has become far more complex. Your successful navigation will be enormously aided by information, by insight into the ways of the system, by a questioning attitude, and by advocacy.

There are five rules for successfully navigating the health care system.

Rule One: Stay Healthy

You will fare better, no matter what your condition, if you take better care of yourself. It seems almost pedestrian to recite the simple things you can do to improve the status of your health, but here they are in case you haven't read a newspaper or watched a television in the past 20 years. First, smoking is actually bad for you. You should quit. The good news is that there are lots of quite effective smoking-cessation aids—everything from the patch to counselling—to get you off the noxious weed. Second, being physically active can reduce your risk of heart disease or cancer. Physical activity could be as easy as walking more or as challenging as going to a gym and working out. Being involved in an active sport will help.

The third in this trinity of things that make you a healthy navigator is what you eat. What you eat is what you are, and there are both good and bad things you can eat. Despite newspaper stories that seem to vacillate on some subjects—for example, whether coffee is good or bad for you—for a long period of time medical evidence has consistently shown the virtues of a balanced diet. There is lots of evidence on the virtues of dark leafy vegetables and an abundant wealth of information on why eating greasy fast food will not increase your health—in fact, it will have the opposite effect.

If you find it hard to believe that fast food is so damaging, take a trip (please walk) to the nearest video store and rent the movie *Super Size Me*. It will likely put you off everything but the salads at McDonald's, Burger King, and Wendy's for the rest of your life. On second thought, be careful of even the salad dressings—the ones at McDonald's contain more fat than the cheeseburgers.

Increasingly, the health care system is trying to save you from yourself and your choices. This is not an act of altruism. Facing rising costs, health care professionals want to postpone your need for treatment for as many years as possible. You can help by staying healthy and making better choices.

Rule Two: Know as Much as You Possibly Can

You need to become informed not only about the condition or disease that you are coping with, but also about the resources in the health system. You need to know how to find care, and find it swiftly. You need to know how to determine if care is safe and high quality. You need to know your insurance coverage, whether that is coverage paid for by your tax dollars through government or supplementary private insurance paid by your employer, or whether you're going to pay out of your own pocket.

You have more and more choices to make, important choices that will affect your health care. You need to know what to expect in your treatment and what you can do to improve your chances of a good outcome. The good news is that this information is often available on the Internet. Because information on the Internet can be disorganized and of uneven quality, you need to separate the good information from the not so good. Today, many reputable organizations and institutions provide basic and reliable information on their websites. Being an informed sailor is the most important rule of navigation, and that rule applies if you're a patient travelling through the health care system. It may be true that ignorance is bliss, but not when it comes to your health or health care. In health care, ignorance can make your patient journey longer and more difficult and your outcome worse.

Just as a good sailor needs to know the winds and currents of the ocean, you need to know the winds and currents of the health system. Having a good knowledge of the health care system, particularly those centres of excellence within it, can be the difference between getting first-class care and waiting a long time for care that wasn't worth the waiting.

Find out what you need and what is covered in your province or territory. Like real estate, health care services have a lot to do with "location, location, location." We often confuse "universality" with "uniformity." We might have a "universal" health care system, in which every resident and citizen is entitled to medicare, but we do not have a system in which the services and products to which we are entitled are the same from coast to coast. Nor is there a guarantee that you will automatically get what you are entitled to receive.

Rule Three: Organize Your Care Team

Your care team will likely start with your family doctor, but as you age, you need to expand that team far beyond just your doctor. Simply finding a family doctor is a challenge for many Canadians. In addition, many of us now take a complex set of medications, so the pharmacist with whom you deal is a vital member of your team. Befriend your pharmacist! A pharmacist is quite capable of being a solid adviser on the use of not only prescription medication but, more important, the over-the-counter remedy that is often the best option for minor ailments. The pharmacist may be your first and only stop for treating minor rashes, illnesses, and aches and pains. However, beyond the physician and pharmacist, you may also need the services of a nurse, nurse-practitioner, dietitian, nutritionist, physiotherapist, or massage therapist. For example, if you are managing lower back pain and wish to avoid surgery that will leave you with a rigid spine, you may need a prescribed set of exercises. The point here is that as medicine and health care become more complex, so does the range of skills you need access to—hence the team! Look to all members of the team for coaching in the management of illness, particularly chronic illness. Remember that you will spend a few hours a year with your team and over 8000 hours a year self-managing your condition.

Rule Four: Have an Advocate

You need someone who is in your corner, particularly if you are dealing with hospitalization or a serious illness. During your patient care journey, you may not always be sufficiently strong or focused or even conscious to deal with what's coming at you. You need someone who has the dual qualities of caring deeply about you and not taking no for an answer. You need your advocate to ask the questions that you may forget to ask. You need your advocate to write down the answers you may forget. In most cases, your advocate will be a family member or close friend. If you do not have a close family member or friend, you may need to seek the support of a professional patient advocate.

Rule Five: Take Control of Your Care—Don't Be a Passive Patient

You need to adopt a questioning, skeptical attitude. Don't presume that all your care providers know your full history. Don't presume they know your allergies. Make a careful point of communicating fully. Often one specialist is unaware that another specialist is treating you with medication, and drugs can interact in negative ways. You need to be in control and keep your care team fully informed.

You also need to own and control your health record. You should not be at the mercy of paper-based medical records systems that make it difficult to retrieve essential test results, X-rays, and other information. Sometimes important records are lost or are not available when needed. Build your own medical record either electronically or in a simple file. Keep track of illnesses, medications, test results, and your family's medical history. You'll learn more about this in Chapter 4.

If you have drawn up an advance directive or living will, you need to ensure all those caring for you are aware of your choices. Only then can you be assured your wishes will be respected and implemented.

Embarking on Your Journey

A few last notes before we take you on a life journey through the Canadian health care system:

This book was created using a mix of information from interviews with leading experts and from some very credible websites. Although good information is accessible through a number of sources, many people don't know where to look and are unsure about how to assess the credibility of what they find. Look up "cancer" with a computer search engine, for example, and you will find websites from reputable, peer-reviewed organizations, but you may also find websites for dishonest organizations professing to cure cancer through a snake oil that you rub on your belly. The purpose of our book is to take what we considered to be important information from credible sources and provide you with a "one-stop shopping place." The resource guides at the end of each chapter highlight the best health-organization websites we have come across, as well as essential books. But there are many other good sources of information—our resource guides are not meant to be exhaustive or exclusive.

This book provides an interpretation of what we, through our own experiences and the experiences of friends, have actually found to be true about the health care system. Where there is evidence, we cite it. Some of you will have had different experiences. Some of the advice we provide may be met with criticism from the "purists" in the health professional community. But these reflect our opinions, and we reserve the right to share them and to pass on some of the tips and tricks we've picked up along the way. This book is meant to provide you with some added practical ammunition for your journey through the health care system in Canada. Your patient care journey will be unique. This book is about helping you to improve that journey.

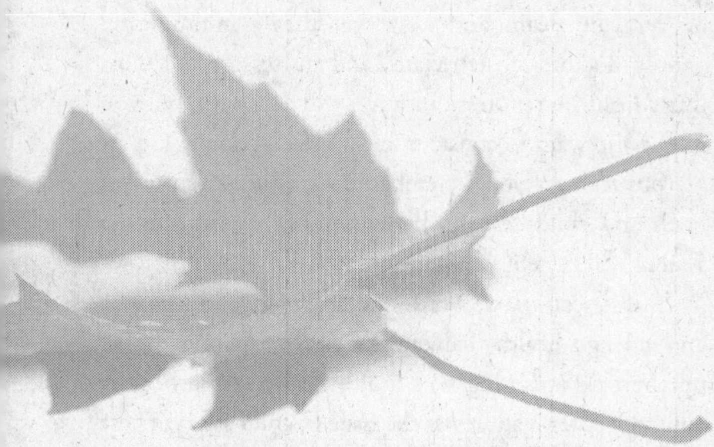

The Early Years

Having a healthy baby and raising a healthy child safely are the shared goals of every parent in Canada. Yet compared to other activities, helping parents seems to fall far down the list of priorities for governments and other organizations. Just think about it—you are required to pass a driving test in order to operate a motor vehicle. Operating a boat in Canada now requires an operator card. Governments promote and provide the means by which we can get the necessary training and licences, and they also emphasize safe driving and safe boating with television ads and printed materials. But when it comes to helping our young mothers and families negotiate the issues of birthing and being a parent, our systems seem disorganized and complex. The choices you will make can be overwhelming—who will be on your team and how will they communicate? Family doctors, obstetricians, and nurses are the most likely front-line professionals you will deal with, but you might also want to consider midwives and doulas as part of your team. If you are embarking on the adventure of birth and child-bearing, knowing how to navigate the system will benefit you and your child.

In this section, we tackle the challenge of pregnancy and having a healthy baby in Chapter 1. Chapter 2 takes up the task of raising that healthy baby into a healthy child. Chapter 3 addresses the issue of child safety. These chapters begin our journey of navigating health and health care.

ONE

Having a Baby in Canada

Many of us remember when family doctors delivered babies. Today, in large urban centres, it seems unusual to have anyone other than a specialist deliver a baby. The Canadian Institute for Health Information (CIHI) confirms this trend. It reports that in 2000, obstetricians performed 61 percent of all vaginal births and 95 percent of all Caesarean births—many more than family physicians. There is also a difference between the city and the country. In urban areas, fewer family doctors (12 percent) deliver babies than family doctors do in small towns and rural areas, where 27 percent perform this service.

Furthermore, it is becoming more frequent for a family doctor to follow the mother only for the first 32 weeks of the pregnancy before transferring her care to other practitioners, including midwives and obstetricians.

The Canadian Institute for Health Information also tells us that

- there are few obstetricians and anaesthetists in remote and rural areas,
- the number of family doctors providing obstetrical services is declining, and
- the number of northern community hospitals that offers obstetrical care has decreased over the past two decades.

A research study cited by CIHI concludes that many family doctors don't want to deliver babies for a number of reasons, including the unpredictable lifestyle that accompanies assisting deliveries. As these doctors know only too well, babies don't necessarily arrive during office hours! Fear of a malpractice suit is another big reason that many family doctors don't want to assist deliveries: There is little wrath or grief to compare to that of a family whose baby has been injured during delivery. Clearly, health system errors are not the only cause of damaged births. Errors have, in fact, lessened. Though the number of malpractice cases launched has decreased, the monetary damages awarded by a court or as a result of a settlement usually are high. It's no surprise, then, that the malpractice insurance fees that doctors who deliver babies pay are high. However, none of this compares with the tragedy faced by a family who has been deprived of an otherwise healthy baby because of a medical error. The burden on the family both emotionally and financially will be an ever-present source of sadness during the child's growth and development.

One American physician advocates bringing a video camera into the delivery room, not only to record what happens during birth but also to act as a powerful record for the future in case of a lawsuit. Although most centres do allow videotaping, mainly as a record of the family bonding with the new baby and to provide some early pictures for the baby album, they require the explicit permission of all health workers in the room at time of birth. However, they will not allow its use for recording monitoring devices or other labour documents such as charts.

There is one other reason that the number of family doctors practising primary-care obstetrics is declining: the absence of system supports. Over the last number of years, as a result of services being rationalized, obstetrical services have been consolidated. That means that fewer smaller hospitals provide the service and most of the care has been transferred to one site. Dr. Michael Helewa, past president of the Society of Obstetricians and Gynecologists of Canada, notes that in his area of Winnipeg over the past 10 years, the number of hospitals offering obstetrical services has been reduced from five to two. This is a common theme across the country. Typically, when a hospital closes its obstetrical service, the family doctors practising in the area tend to stop assisting deliveries rather than arranging to transfer their hospital privileges to another hospital, which may be much farther away.

When we consider that specialists are scarce and family doctors are reducing their obstetrical practices, we see a troubling trend, especially if you live outside an urban centre. To get the care you need, you may have to be transferred to an urban centre. Having a baby closer to home is easier for urban Canadians than it is for rural Canadians.

As you navigate your way through the channels of the health care system, remember that this journey is a very different one than it was even a few years ago, as the statistics cited above suggest. To help you, this chapter will look at the resources available to expectant parents, emerging resources, who does what, and what you can expect within the context of somewhat limited access to people who can help you deliver a healthy baby in Canada.

Let's look at the team that will care for you throughout your pregnancy: doctors, nurses, midwives, and various technicians.

Doctors

According to data compiled by CIHI, the majority of family doctors who practise primary maternity care provide "shared care." This means they follow the mother for a certain amount of time before the delivery and then transfer her care to a midwife, an obstetrician, or another family doctor who does obstetrics. If your doctor is part of a group practice, your baby might be delivered by a doctor from the group and not your regular doctor. Not all obstetrician/gynecologists (OBGYN) do obstetrics. The Society of Gynecology and Obstetrics estimates that only a little over 50 percent of all OBGYNs practise primary maternity care.

To assist in delivering babies, doctors must have hospital privileges. They are usually affiliated with one hospital, so you will need to deliver your baby in that hospital. Because it is important that you are as comfortable and confident with the facility as you are with your doctor, be sure you know which hospital your family doctor is affiliated with and whether that hospital promotes moral attitudes contrary to your own. For example, should your test results indicate a severe birth defect that would cause you personally to decide to terminate your pregnancy, you will need to know that your doctor or your hospital will manage your situation in a way that is acceptable to you. Although many people have argued that the doctor will defend the hospital where he or she has privileges and thus is not the best person to ask, most doctors are very ethical people. If they know a given place has particular policies or moral attitudes and you ask the question directly, you are likely to get an honest answer. More important, any ethical doctor, regardless of personal or religious beliefs, will facilitate your decisions by organizing your transfer to another facility should such a request arise. They will help navigate your care.

Choosing a Doctor When You Are Having a Baby

The comedian Jackie Mason has a most wonderful and relevant joke: "He's terrific! Fantastic! The best doctor in New York! He's so great (pause) you'll never get in to see him!" In Chapter 4, we discuss some of the general considerations that go into choosing a family doctor. Two of the biggies are experience and access.

Family doctors practising primary maternity care have training and the experience required, though there is a shortage of family doctors who practise this kind of medicine. If you are under the care of an obstetrician, he or she will have the required training and experience.

It is really crucial to find a doctor who is accessible and has either a group practice or nurses in the practice to support the doctor when he or she is not available to see or speak to you.

Given the shortage of doctors who practise primary maternity care, your ability to choose a doctor may be limited. And even where there is a good doctor (family or specialist), typically he or she is so booked up that you may feel a successful appointment is conducted in sound bites. Generally, though, your care provider (family doctor or nurse-practitioner) will help you navigate to someone who does primary maternity care.

If you are lucky enough to live in an area with enough doctors to offer a choice, take into account the type of facilities the doctors have and how close you are to their office. Some doctors have ultrasound facilities close by. Proximity to the doctor and to the nearest ultrasound services will be very convenient when you are pregnant. If tests are required you will not have to travel far to get to an ultrasound clinic.

Questions to Ask

- What supports does your doctor provide after hours?
- Is he or she part of an on-call group?
- Does he or she have a nurse answer the phone?
- What is the after-hours phone number?
- What supports does your doctor have during office hours?
- Does your doctor have a nurse on site in case he or she is not immediately available?
- Are there testing facilities close by (ultrasounds, for example)?
- If something goes wrong, what do you do?
- Where will you deliver and who will deliver the baby?
- If your doctor practises in a group, be sure you are comfortable with the group practice approach. Ask your doctor whether he or she will deliver your baby or if it might be someone else. Some mothers find it unsettling to see a new face in the delivery room when they were not expecting it. Also, ask your doctor about the rest of the group, who's in it and what kind of support you can expect from them.
- Check that the hospital in which your doctor helps deliver your baby has a good reputation for birth deliveries, that it is equipped to deal with emergencies, and that it does not promote moral attitudes contrary to your own.

Dealing with Doctors When You Are Having a Baby

In Chapter 4, we provide some tips on how to maximize your visit with the doctor. Here are some that you should know when you are having a baby:

- Before your first visit to your doctor to discuss your pregnancy, get a good book on the subject. Several excellent books are listed in the Resource Guide at the end of this chapter.
- Compile your list of questions between appointments as issues come up and take notes at your appointments. *Do not* wait until the night before to try to remember your questions—chances are, you won't be able to summon them. Leaving out the details of a symptom might have significant implications on your care. Francesca's obstetrician had a busy practice. At each appointment he had a clear agenda of the items he needed to discuss but if she didn't also arrive with a list of questions, the interview became quite one-sided. Francesca learned quickly to tell him immediately that she had questions written down. He would listen to all questions and answer. Sometimes, he would check things out as a result of an issue that was raised. In addition, she wrote down all his answers because often the same things would worry her again and she would have trouble remembering his exact response. It was very comforting to go back and read his point-form answers.

- Manage your expectations about the amount of time a doctor will give a patient who is low risk and doing fine. Most books talk about finding a doctor you can "talk to" but what you talk about is important too. If you have a question, an issue, a problem, or a concern directly related to your condition, you do need to be able to relate well to your doctor. But if "talk" means sharing with the doctor your knowledge about the developmental phases of a fetus, for example, a doctor with a waiting room full of patients may get a little edgy. We make this point again in Chapter 4. Many obstetricians or family doctors who practise primary maternity care have nurse-practitioners who will provide support and answers to many of your questions.

Questions to Ask

What over-the-counter medicines can I still take for:

- Fever
- Upset stomach
- Headache

Nurses

Nurses can provide many services to pregnant mothers. They include the following:

- Childbirth education
- Pre-birth counselling

- Home-care services
- Assisting labour and delivery

Some nurses are also qualified to provide lactation consulting.

You might also have a nurse-practitioner as part of your team. Nurse-practitioners are nurses with special additional training that allows them to undertake some clinical services that doctors normally provide. They can order certain tests, diagnose certain conditions, and prescribe some medications. In most provinces, nurse-practitioners are allowed to practise on their own without a doctor. However, the clinical services they are allowed to provide, regardless of their training, is dependent on where they practise in Canada.

Nurses are often indispensable to a physician practice. Dr. Michael Helewa is a firm believer in the "team" concept of delivering care. He has nurse-practitioners, nurses, and midwives all working together at Saint Boniface Hospital in Winnipeg. The team approach to primary maternity care is becoming more popular in Canada. By the time Dr. Helewa walks into the examining room, the expectant mother has already had a visit with a nurse, who will have answered many, if not most, of her questions. Nurses provide both clinical support and coaching and are often better than doctors at it. As Dr. Paul Wallace from Kaiser Permanente, a U.S. not-for-profit health care organization, said in a recent conference in Toronto, "Doctors like to think they are great coaches, but they are actually lousy at coaching; nurses do a much better job."

Anaesthesiologists (and Epidurals)

We know of a family doctor who, when asked by his patient whether she should have an epidural, given that she wanted to have a "natural childbirth," responded, "All childbirth is natural. Will that be with or without pain?"

Epidural anaesthesia is used in 35 percent of births in Canada to provide pain relief during labour and delivery and is administered by specialists called anaesthesiologists. They also may provide neonatal resuscitation. Small and rural hospitals may not offer epidurals because they need to be administered by an anaesthesiologist and require specialized resuscitation equipment, which smaller hospitals may not have. Family doctors may also give epidurals. Ask your caregiver (doctor, nurse-practitioner, or midwife) whether your hospital offers epidurals.

There are many horror stories of badly administered epidurals. Some books will tell you that you are wise to ask for the staff anaesthesiologist and not a resident, who would have less experience. However, in the hospital, the wait for the staff anaesthesiologist may be long and you may never get your epidural because he or she is busy. How big a problem is this? Junior residents do not give epidurals on their own—they need supervision by a staff anaesthesiologist. Senior residents may proceed with an epidural but with the permission of the attending or staff anaesthesiologist. Still, it is wise to ask how many epidurals the resident has administered. If you are in a hospital that delivers a lot of babies, there is a good chance that the senior resident is every bit as good as the staff anaesthesiologist and has lots of experience. After all, that is what you are looking for, experience. Practice makes perfect in medical care as well as other endeavours.

If you have decided in advance that you do not want to have an epidural, ask your doctor what to do and who to speak to if you change your mind. It is also good to know whether there is a point beyond which an epidural should not be given and what that is.

Ultrasound Technicians and Ultrasounds

Ultrasounds have become one of the most commonplace tests undertaken during a pregnancy. The job of the ultrasound technician is to administer the test by scanning your abdomen. The technician's job ends there. Yes, these tests are considered safe but they are tests nonetheless. The validity of the test is in the interpretation of the results. Although ultrasound technicians are incredibly well trained and know how to read an ultrasound very well, they don't have access to certain information, nor are they trained to diagnose. A trained person—usually your family doctor or obstetrician—must read and interpret the results. If the results are not well read or not read within the context of other tests or clinical findings, you can be given a false sense of security. An ultrasound alone does not provide for a complete diagnosis and the technician does not have access to this other relevant information.

A technician can show you the heartbeat during a routine ultrasound as he or she is taking fetal measurements. But if the doctor is worried about something and needs answers, a trained physician must view the film, assess other information, and report back. This is often unpopular with worried expectant mothers. Many ultrasound techs have suffered tongue lashings at the hands of mothers desperate to know the outcome of these tests. This is understandable. But it is not fair to the technician and it is not good medicine.

Two things that an ultrasound clinic must have are the following:

- Certification that it meets standards in your jurisdiction
- Certified physicians to read the results

Some ultrasound clinics will provide, for a fee, a 3D picture of your baby. These services are not for the purpose of diagnosing problems, though—they are basic photo ops for your unborn child. Many members of the medical profession frown on the use of these tests for reasons other than monitoring the baby. Ultrasounds use energy waves that produce heat. Subjecting the baby to any interventions for purposes other than diagnosis is generally not a good idea.

Midwives

Many women reportedly prefer midwives because they feel that these practitioners will take more time with them. Midwives have a knowledge of obstetrics and provide care for women in all stages of pregnancy, including labour, childbirth, and postpartum care up to six weeks after the baby is born. As CIHI reports, regulated midwives (and to some extent unregulated midwives) can and do help deliver babies just like a doctor. Where there are complicating factors, you will require medical help from a doctor.

Until the early 1990s Canada was one of a few countries that did not have midwifery legislation. However, this service is now regulated in most parts of Canada. What does regulation mean? Regulated midwives can prescribe certain medicines and they can order appropriate tests during pregnancy. However, regulation of midwifery does not automatically mean that these services are covered by public insurance in every province and territory. And where they are allowed to deliver babies (at home, in hospitals, or in birthing centres) also differs from coast to coast.

In Canada midwives are registered with and regulated by the College of Midwives of their province. There is no national regulatory body for midwifery. As a result, there is quite a patchwork of regulation and funding for midwifery across the country. Some provinces still do not have legislation for midwives. In some provinces, practising midwives do not have

Tip

If you have chosen to use the services of a regulated midwife and you want to know about a possible birth defect, make sure you request the appropriate test. Doctors will usually automatically offer you that choice. Regulated midwives may not.

hospital privileges. In other jurisdictions, midwifery services are not funded and women who want to use a midwife must pay for it themselves. Training requirements also vary from province to province and, therefore, so too do the services that midwives are permitted to perform. In some provinces, they can assist births in hospitals just like doctors. In others, they provide mostly support and education throughout the pregnancy, birth, and post-birth period. It is very important that you consult the website of the Canadian Association of Midwives (CAM), listed in the Resource section, to find up-to-date information regarding the regulation, legislation, and funding of midwives in your province or territory.

The chart below shows these cross-country discrepancies as they existed in 2004.

Although more women are reportedly choosing midwives to deliver their babies, it would appear that the vast majority of these births are also physician assisted. Midwifery is not supported very well in Canada. Midwives are only allowed to have 50 to 60 clients annually in some jurisdictions, making it difficult for it

Midwifery Across Canada

Province/ Territory	Legislation (Year)	Funded	Out-of-Pocket Payment	Home, Hospital, or Birth Centre	Midwifery School
B.C.	Yes (1998)	Yes	No	Home/hospital	Yes
Alta.	Yes (1996)	No	Yes	Home/hospital/ birth centre	No
Sask.	Yes (act not yet proclaimed)	No	Yes	Home	No
Man.	Yes (2000)	Yes	No	Home/hospital	No
Ont.	Yes (1994)	Yes	No	Home/hospital	Yes
Que.	Yes (1999)	Yes	No	Birth centre (soon to be expanded to home and a few hospitals)	Yes
N.B.	No	No	Yes	Home	No
N.S.	No	No	Yes	Home	No
P.E.I.	No	No	Yes	Home	No
N.L.	No	No	No	Hospital (remote areas only)	No
Y.T.	No	No	Yes	Home	No
N.W.T.	Yes (act to be proclaimed in 2004)	Yes (2004)	Yes (before 2004)	Home	No
Nun.	Partially (one pilot project in Rankin Inlet)	Partially	No	Birth centre	No

Source: Canadian Institute for Health Information, *Giving Birth in Canada*, 2004, p. 11.

to be a viable profession. Furthermore, very few schools that train midwives exist in Canada.

A number of Canadian and international studies suggest that there is a difference in the type of care provided by family doctors, obstetricians, and midwives. CIHI gives a detailed account of the studies in "Giving Birth in Canada" (2004). The highlights of these studies show that women cared for by midwives generally

- had fewer tests, such as ultrasounds, genetic amniocentesis, and glucose screening;
- were less likely to be hospitalized prenatally, to undergo a Caesarean section, and to give birth to preterm babies;
- were less likely to receive an epidural;
- were less likely to have their labour induced; and
- were less likely to have an episiotomy.

Tip

Episiotomies are incisions made to the opening of the vagina during the late stages of labour. The practice was based on the belief that a clean, controlled cut will reduce tearing, which could bring on complications later. According to recent studies, episiotomies do not protect mothers from severe tears. The practice of routine episiotomy has been abolished in this country. However, this procedure may have to be done under certain circumstances.

These findings are not totally surprising. Patients who are also high risk and for whom these interventions are needed are those most frequently under the care of a doctor.

Doulas

A doula is a woman who is trained and experienced in birth support and provides birth support services and/or postpartum services, though she is usually not a nurse. She is independent and self-employed. She provides support to the mother and her partner during pregnancy, labour, birth, and the postpartum period. She offers emotional support (reassurance, perspective, and encouragement), physical comfort (breathing techniques, positioning and movement, touch and massage, relaxation techniques, etc.), and informational and interpretive support to assist her clients to make informed decisions about their care. A doula does not offer medical choices or options. A doula is employed by you and helps promote the birth you desire. She will assist you and your partner in preparing your birth plan. A birth doula can accompany you to the hospital when you have your baby and will provide support during the birthing process.

Before heading into a hospital with a doula to have your baby, try to find out if the hospital is "doula friendly." Some doulas feel that some hospital nurses frown on their presence.

A doula does not deliver babies, perform clinical tasks (blood pressures, fetal heart tones, vaginal exams), give medical advice, or interfere with the advice given by your care provider. She does not take over the role of your primary support person (unless requested) but helps to guide him or her.

Tip

Ask your doctor or midwife about the hospital in which you will deliver and whether doulas fare well in that setting. Check with some friends who had a doula and who delivered in that hospital. And check with the doula! They know when and where they are welcome.

Doulas are *not* midwives—their training typically consists of two- to three-day seminars provided by two certifying organizations: Doulas of North America (DONA) and the Childbirth and Postpartum Professional Association. The websites listed in the Resources section will describe the certifying criteria and will also list training dates and locations.

According to some research, women who work with a doula have 26 percent less chance of a Caesarean birth; have 28 percent less need for epidurals or analgesics (when desired); have a higher success rate of Vaginal Birth After C-Section (VBAC); have 41 percent less need for assisted birth; are 33 percent less likely to have negative feelings about their birth experience; and tend to have a more nurturing attitude toward their baby.

Postpartum doulas are becoming a popular addition to doula care. This type of doula provides support to new parents in the first few days or weeks at home by

- reassurance, support, teaching, and education concerning infant care (feeding, sleeping, bathing,

etc.) and the new mother's care (eating well, getting enough rest, postpartum adjustment, etc.),
- assistance with light housekeeping (laundry, shopping, meal preparation) if required.

Tip

Do not hire a doula if you are hoping for help making medical, clinical, or moral decisions regarding your pregnancy or your child. A doula will obtain information to help you make informed decisions, but she will not and should not make decisions for you.

Interview two or three doulas to find the one who best suits you and your partner—after all, you will probably be spending a fair bit of time with her!

Request references or ask friends for referrals.

Ask your caregiver about his or her experience with doulas and also if the hospital welcomes the presence of doulas.

Doulas are self-employed and each offers different experience and training—ask for their contracts and fees.

Doulas will not provide decision support on clinical matters, medical matters, or moral issues.

They will not answer questions such as "I am five days overdue and the doctor wants to induce me on Tuesday, which will be seven days overdue. Should I say okay?" or "They want to break my water. What do you think?" There have been cases in which doulas have resigned from a case, having been put under great pressure to answer questions or help make decisions outside their mandate. This can be traumatic for the expectant mother.

What Tests Will You Be Given?

The Society of Obstetricians and Gynecologists of Canada recommends a prenatal visit every 4 to 6 weeks until about 28 to 30 weeks and then every 2 to 3 until 36 weeks. After that, the visits are recommended to take place every 1 to 2 weeks until delivery.

In addition to the schedule of routine visits with the doctor, women in Canada do receive a great deal of information on a number of important topics such as nutrition, exercise and breastfeeding, labour and delivery, as well as other important information about the pregnancy, the kinds of tests that will be required and why, and optional tests.

A good resource book about pregnancy can provide you with the details on what these tests involve and what they test for. It should also provide you with a comprehensive description for the various conditions or risks that these tests can identify.

The routine care for pregnant mothers that is covered by your provincial or territorial insurance plan includes the following:

- Pregnancy test
- Medical history (both yours and relevant family history)
- Full physical checkup and internal physical exam of the reproductive organs and pelvis (the mother's weight and blood pressure are also taken for comparison purposes)

- Blood tests for
    - Rh blood type
    - CBC (complete blood count)
    - Blood sugar level
    - Immunity to rubella (German measles), varicella (chickenpox), syphilis, and hepatitis B
- Cultures for sexually transmitted diseases
- Multiple serum screening for trisomies and anomalies (birth defects)
- Urine tests
- Pap test
- Ultrasound scanning

Depending on the circumstances of the mother, a doctor may order additional tests or examinations, all of which are covered by provincial and territorial drug plans; an example of an additional test is HIV screening in pregnancy (antiretroviral treatment can be effective in stopping the mother-to-child transmission).

Some tests that screen for birth defects can be done before a child is even conceived. When the doctor feels there is a risk that a potential mother may be a carrier for certain diseases, the expectant mother is tested at the expense of the provincial or territorial plan. Some examples of diseases that a woman can be screened for are

- Cystic fibrosis
- Sickle-cell anemia

- Tay-Sachs disease
- Thalassemia

If you are worried about being a carrier of one of these disorders, you should talk to your doctor before getting pregnant. He or she can then decide on your risk factor and test you if it is appropriate.

Once you are pregnant, a number of tests can be offered to ensure that your baby does not have a birth defect. These tests differ in accuracy and risk. One test, maternal serum screening (MSS), is very safe—it is done on a blood sample—and is becoming more common in Canada. The test looks for different "markers" that are analyzed, and results determine the rate of risk for birth defect and genetic anomalies. MSS tests are made up of single, double, and triple screening; recently quadruple screening has been introduced. The more screening that is conducted on the samples, the greater the chance of reducing the false positive and thus lessening the need for invasive testing. However, MSS tests are funded to different degrees across the country. Only British Columbia, Saskatchewan, Manitoba, Ontario, and Newfoundland and Labrador cover the "triple-screen test," which offers a more refined estimate of risk. All jurisdictions cover the single-screen test but it is not as accurate. You can opt to pay for more screening yourself. The Society of Obstetricians and Gynaecologists of Canada estimates that the out-of-pocket cost to a woman paying for the double-screen test is about $40 and the triple-screen test is $80 (figures current in 2006). You will want to consider getting a triple-screen test done if you are concerned about birth defects, even if it isn't covered in your jurisdiction, because of its greater accuracy. Don't forget to find out if your employer's benefit plan will reimburse you if it is not covered by your province or territory.

Amniocentesis and chorionic villus sampling, which test for birth defects, are covered by all jurisdictions for women who are either over 35, have a history of birth defects, or have been identified as high risk due to the results of other tests like ultrasound. These tests are not covered by provincial and territorial health plans for women who do not fit these categories. Note too that these tests carry with them their own risks such as a miscarriage or birth defect.

Birth Plans

During the course of your visits, members of your caregiver team (doctor, nurse, midwife, or doula) may encourage you to fill out a birth plan. This plan will give direction on what your wishes are—for example:

- Whether you want medication
- Which interventions, if any, are acceptable to you
- Who you want in the room with you

Midwives, doulas, and doctors or hospitals will either provide you with a form that you fill in or work with you to create one. Check around for ideas on what to include in your birth plan. Talk to friends about what they have included.

Francesca was offered the option of having an amniocentesis when she was pregnant and over 35. Her concerns about the safety of the test were allayed when the doctor told her that he'd never had a patient miscarry in 10 years. No one will tell you that the test is without risk, but the experience of the people doing it and that of the place you are having it done are very important factors.

Hospital Choices and Length of Stay

If you are like many women in Canada, chances are you don't have much choice regarding where you deliver your baby. But if you do have some choice, here are some things you will want to consider:

- Does the hospital have high volumes of delivery? (Higher is usually better.)
- In a low-volume hospital, is there neonatal support if there is a problem with the birth? Can you be easily transferred to a more specialized setting if there is a problem? Are the doctors and nurses on site trained in neonatal resuscitation?
- In a low-volume hospital, does your physician have access to specialists for consultation?
- What kind of facilities does the hospital have for giving birth—are there birthing rooms, birth chairs, etc.?

- Is the hospital doula friendly?
- Is the hospital "baby friendly"?

"Baby friendly" is a designation created by the World Health Organization and UNICEF, and given to hospitals with practices that promote and support breastfeeding. In 2003, CIHI reported that only two hospitals in Canada had this status. By 2006 the number had doubled, and two community health centres had been added. (See the Resources section at the end of this chapter.) Even without the designation, many hospitals do promote and provide some support for breastfeeding. The Breastfeeding Committee for Canada recommends that all staff dealing with pregnant or breastfeeding mothers should have at least 18 hours of training in this field. You may hear it referred to as the "18-hour course." If it is important to you, ask if the hospital has adopted this practice of training its staff.

The average hospital stay for a healthy woman having an uncomplicated delivery is 24 to 48 hours, but the length of stay varies across Canada. The jurisdictions with the shortest length of stay for vaginal deliveries without any instruments are Alberta, Ontario, and Nunavut. The longest length of stay for the same type of births tends to be in eastern Canada. Clearly, if there are complications, the stay is longer. However, consider that 20 years ago, women often stayed in the hospital close to five days for an uncomplicated birth. The CIHI data show that with the shorter hospital stays, there is a higher readmission rate for newborns suffering from jaundice.

The data also show that a greater number of babies in Canada are arriving either prematurely or before the due date. This trend is found not only in Canada but elsewhere and is often attributed to the increased number of twins and triplets as a consequence of advanced reproductive technology.

Earlier discharge is not necessarily a bad thing if everything is going well. However, there are situations where an extra day or two can make all the difference, as Francesca found out. When she was in hospital for the birth of her child, Ontario was in the grip of the SARS epidemic (so no visitors were allowed), her husband had been hospitalized for weeks for a serious health problem and she had not been allowed to see him (also because of SARS), and her father was dying in Sudbury, a city about 250 miles (400 km) north of Toronto, where she lived.

She decided to try to stay as long as possible in the hospital, where she would have food and care and support during this difficult time. But hospitals have their timelines, and if your baby is born normally without complication and you are deemed healthy—both of which applied to Francesca—then you are out. Full stop. However, as she told her obstetrician about her situation, Francesca burst into tears. He told her not to worry and said that he would deal with it.

She was able to stay a little longer, and she found those few more days made the difference between coping and not coping. When she did request that she be discharged, she felt more confident and wasn't feeling like someone was throwing her from a train!

Tip

If you are undergoing a tough situation at home and you really need a little extra time, the best advocate in this case is not your mother, your husband, or your great-aunt Gertrude (convincing though she may be). Talk to your doctor. That is the person who can judge the situation best and, if he or she feels it warrants it, intervene on your behalf. Your doctor will have pull in the hospital, but you probably don't.

Having Baby at Home versus in the Hospital

The debate over home versus hospital deliveries has been raging for a long time and is not going to go away any time soon. There are some important issues to weigh if you are undecided about the best place for your delivery. If you are interested in having a baby at home, you should be assisted by a registered midwife to lower your risk, but you should also know that epidurals cannot be given at home. If you are sure that you want an epidural, you must deliver in a medical centre. Also, doctors do not deliver babies at home.

According to Statistics Canada data reported by CIHI, 99 percent of babies in Canada are born in hospitals. Recently, a large study conducted in the United

States and Canada by Kenneth C. Johnson and Betty-Anne Daviss concluded that low-risk, at-home births are as safe as and more convenient than hospital births. The study compared at-home, low-risk births to low-risk hospital births (assisted by qualified practitioners—doctors and midwives) and found the following about rates of interventions:

- Five percent of the women at home needed epidurals, compared to 63 percent in hospital; in Canada, epidurals are not allowed to be given at home.
- Two percent of the home-birth women needed episiotomies, compared to 33 percent in hospital.
- Forceps were needed for 1 percent of at-home women, compared to 2 percent in hospital.
- Five times fewer at-home women delivered with Caesarean sections in the event of an emergency, compared to hospital rates.
- The rate of infant deaths was similar to those delivered in hospital.
- About 12 percent of women who wanted to give birth at home had to be taken to hospital because of complications or pain.

Co-author Betty-Anne Daviss writes that "the risk for home births is very similar to hospital birth, but you have one-tenth to one-half the intervention, so a lot of the caesareans being done, a lot of the forceps being done in hospital, are not really necessary."

The study is gaining a great deal of attention around the world on an issue that remains very controversial. On one side of the debate, many women and health care providers such as midwives have felt that home birth for low-risk cases is both natural and favourable. The study seems to support this position.

However, many argue that having a baby at home is risky because something can go wrong even if mother and baby are healthy and the delivery is expected to be uncomplicated. The Society of Obstetricians and Gynaecologists of Canada is concerned that although many births may take place without problems, when there *is* a problem, things can deteriorate very quickly. It also points out that a home environment, while comforting, may actually interfere with the ability of the woman to get immediate care.

Bear in mind that 98 percent of the data in this study came from the United States and only 2 percent from Canada. The United States tends to have higher intervention rates in hospitals than Canada, so the data may not correspond well to what is going on here, and the sample in Canada is too small to be significant.

In addition, the researchers compared "low risk" in both home births and hospitals. But on closer examination, "low risk," as they defined it, could include a lot of women who are actually higher risk by other definitions. And these women tend to deliver in hospital. For example, according to the study, low-risk women were those who delivered the child at term (not premature), had a spontaneous birth (not induced), and had a baby that presented with its head first (not a breech). Any birth that met these three criteria was included in both hospital births and home births for the purpose of the study.

But women who had hypertension or diabetes, for example, conditions that could have serious repercussions on risk during birth, would have been included in their definition of "low-risk." Women in this category would have almost certainly been advised to give birth in a hospital rather than at home. Therefore, we believe the sample is somewhat compromised.

Epidurals cannot be administered at home. Women who prefer to give birth at home are generally women who tend not to want any external intervention, including chemical pain management. So it is not surprising that the number of epidurals needed by women giving birth at home is so low.

The debate will continue for a long time to come. There are examples of increased risk on both sides. Those who argue against home delivery could present a case such as this: A baby is being delivered in a home many kilometres from a hospital. The cord is prolapsed (which means that the cord starts coming out before the presenting part of the baby). The baby pushing up against the prolapsed cord can squeeze off its own supply of blood and oxygen, a very serious condition that may even lead to severe brain damage or death. The timeline for help is variable but can be terribly short. A call to 911 will not usually be sufficient, and the results may be tragic.

Those on the other side would argue that medical errors are committed in hospitals when births are rushed—something, they would say, that is much less likely at home (a claim we cannot substantiate). Both sides can present statistics to support their view. And in the end, it is a personal decision that should be based on knowledge of your own condition, the condition of your baby, your medical team, and the plans in place in case of an emergency. We believe this last concern is lessened greatly by choosing hospital deliveries.

Infertility

Experts consider a couple to be infertile when they are unable to conceive after trying for one year. In 2004, Health Canada in its on-line report "Assisted Human Reproduction at Health Canada" estimated that about one in eight Canadian couples experiences infertility.

CIHI reports that most jurisdictions in Canada will cover tests that can help reveal the reason that a couple may be having difficulty conceiving—for example, semen analysis. Also, many jurisdictions will cover some corrective treatment such as repairs to varicoceles and fallopian tubes or endometriosis cauterization.

If you require assisted reproductive technology (ART), these methods are not fully covered by provincial or territorial health plans. Ontario covers limited in vitro fertilization. A great debate is raging over whether assisted reproductive technologies should be publicly funded—ARTs can be very expensive. The question of whether a government should cover some of the cost of ART has resulted in Charter challenges in Ontario and Nova Scotia. However, the court decided in both cases that the provinces had the jurisdiction to choose, restrict, or deny coverage of some ARTs.

The most common reproductive technologies being used in Canada are

- In vitro fertilization (IVF) and intracytoplasmic sperm injection (ICSI)
- Artificial insemination

As of 2006, Ontario is the only province that funds IVF, but it does so only for women with completely blocked fallopian tubes. IVF/ICSI treatment can cost thousands of dollars and the price varies depending on the clinic in which it is done. Our Resources section lists the Canadian Fertility and Andrology Society, which will provide useful information on the subject as well as a listing of IVF clinics in Canada.

A common thread to all the information provided is the following: The place where you have your baby is as important as the emotional support and medical assistance you seek. A hospital may or may not have moral positions on certain matters. It may or may not be doula friendly or baby friendly. It may be a place where lots of babies are born or it may not be such a place. These things are important, some more than others.

If you are embarking on an interaction with the Canadian health care system to have a baby, you need to know yourself, and what you want. You need to manage your expectations and help yourself by being prepared when you see your doctor.

Did You Know?

Rates for assisted delivery using forceps or vacuum extraction tend to be higher in East Coast provinces.

"Caesarean on demand" is a recent phenomenon. This is the practice of booking a Caesarean section without any medical reason.

Some women favour this practice rather than going through the vaginal birth process. But, as with any intervention, there is increased risk. The Society for Obstetricians and Gynaecologists of Canada has issued a position statement against Caesarean section on demand. If you have had a Caesarean section in the past, this does not necessarily mean that you cannot give birth vaginally in subsequent deliveries.

RESOURCE GUIDE

BOOKS

Healthy Beginnings, Third Edition. A. B. Lalonde and Nan Schuurmans (Toronto: Society of Obstetricians and Gynaecologists of Canada, 2006).

What to Expect When You're Expecting. Heidi Murkoff and Sharon Mazel (New York: Simon & Schuster Ltd., 2006).

What to Expect: Eating Well When You're Expecting. Heidi Murkoff and Sharon Mazel (New York: Workman Publishing Co., 2005).

1,000 Questions about Your Pregnancy. Jeffrey Thurston (Irving, Texas: Tapestry Press, 2002).

All these books are exceptional. They walk you through a great deal of information in a very readable way and are recommended by many nurses and physicians. Any of them will serve you well as your reference book throughout pregnancy.

Healthy Beginnings is the only purely Canadian resource of its kind. At about $20, it provides great value and it is now available from Indigo, Chapters, and Coles. It can also be ordered through the Society of Obstetricians and Gynaecologists of Canada.

WEBSITES

"Outcomes of Planned Home Births with Certified Professional Midwives: Large Prospective Study in North America." Kenneth C. Johnson and Betty-Anne Daviss: 2005.

You can read the study results for this paper by going to http://bmj.bmjjournals.com/cgi/content/abstract/330/7505/1416 or simply go to the *British Medical Journal*'s website at www.bmj.com and search for planned home births.

Web MD
www.webmd.com
This website is a terrific resource to look up general medical information on conditions. An area called Pregnancy and Family includes a week-by-week guide to your pregnancy.

ORGANIZATIONS AND ASSOCIATIONS

Society of Obstetricians and Gynaecologists of Canada
www.sogc.org
Telephone: 1-800-561-2416
This website provides information on women's health, including menopause, pregnancy, and general women's health issues. It also provides up-to-date position statements from the organization on a number of issues that you may find interesting.

Canadian Fertility and Andrology Society
www.cfas.ca
Telephone: (514) 524-9009
This organization offers a great listing of fertility clinics in Canada.

Canadian Association of Midwives
www.canadianmidwives.org
Telephone: (514) 807-3668
The best feature on this website for women interested in knowing about the services provided in their own province or territory is the "Across Canada" link. Click

on it and then on the jurisdiction in which you live to get information on the status and regulation of programs in your jurisdiction. There is also contact information about other programs.

Childbirth and Postpartum Professional Association
www.cappa.net
This organization certifies doulas and its website has a resource for finding a doula.

Doula Care
www.doulacare.ca
Telephone: (905) 842-3385 (for the Greater Toronto Area) or 1-888-879-3199 (for all other areas)
This organization is the Canadian association for doulas and will provide you with listings for doulas as well as information about doula care, including the questions you should ask.

DONA International
www.dona.org
DONA International is the international association for doulas. It provides general information and the website allows you to access doula support in your jurisdiction. Also certifies doulas.

Motherisk
www.motherisk.org
Telephone:
1-877-327-4636: Alcohol and Substance Abuse
1-800-436-8477: Nausea and Vomiting
1-888-246-5840: HIV and HIV Treatment
(416) 813-6780: Motherisk's Home Line
Motherisk is run from the Hospital for Sick Children in Toronto. It is a service that is available to all Canadian mothers. Motherisk provides authoritative information and guidance to pregnant or lactating patients and their health care providers regarding the fetal risks associated with infection, disease, and drug, chemical, or radiation exposure(s) during pregnancy. It can help answer questions such as "What can I safely take if I have a terrible headache?"

BABY FRIENDLY HOSPITALS AND BIRTHING CENTRES IN CANADA

For the complete list of all officially designated baby-friendly hospitals and community health centres in Canada, go to The Breastfeeding Committee for Canada website at http://breastfeedingcanada.ca.

At the top left, find Baby Friendly Initiativc, then Canadian Facilities Designated as Baby-Friendly PDF (updated).

For more about the WHO/UNICEF Baby-Friendly Initiative (BFI) go to www.breastfeedingalberta.ca/baby-friendly_initiative.htm.

Installation Hôpital Brome-Missisquoi-Perkins du Centre de santé et de services sociaux la Pommeraie
Website: www.hopitalbmp.qc.ca/
Telephone: (450) 266-5503
950, rue Principale
Cowansville, Quebec J2K 1K3

St. Joseph's Healthcare Hamilton
Website: www.stjoes.ca/default.asp
Telephone: (905) 522-4941
50 Carlton Avenue E.
Hamilton, Ontario L8N 4A6

For a more complete list of Maison de naissance in Quebec, go to www.mimosa.qc.ca/coordonnees_mdn.html

Centre hospitalier Saint-Eustache
Website: www.moncsss.com
Telephone: (450) 473-6811, ext. 2185
520, boul. Arthur-Sauvé
Saint-Eustache, Quebec J7R 5B1

Maison de naissance Mimosa du Centre de santé et de services sociaux du Grand Littoral
Website: www.mimosa.qc.ca
Telephone: (418) 839-0205
182, rue de l'Église
Saint-Romuald, Quebec G6W 3G9

Baby Friendly Community Health Services in Canada
Mission communautaire du Centre de santé et de services sociaux d'Argenteuil
Telephone: (450) 562-4711, ext. 8237
145, avenue de la Providence
Lachute, Quebec J8H 4C7

Mission communautaire du Centre de santé et de services sociaux de CLSC La Pommeraie
Telephone: (450) 266-2522
112, rue Sud
Cowansville, Quebec J2K 2X2

TWO

Getting the Best Care for Your Child

The Hospital for Sick Children in Toronto boasts a cheerful and airy atrium complete with a "Main Street" lined with cafés, stores, and displays. Great big elevators like rockets shoot up and down the walls of the atrium, carrying passengers to floors that look out over the huge entrance. Large puppets perched up high in the air smile down on the tiny visitors below. For many kids, this is home—at least for a while. The lobby exudes activity, joy, and hope. The reality facing many children and parents entering this building is often quite different. Children and their parents, from all over Canada and the world, make the journey to be treated in this state-of-the-art facility. And the hospital has spared no creativity to make the patients' stay as hopeful and positive an experience as it can be.

When Francesca met with Dr. Marvin Gans, a leading Canadian pediatrician at Toronto's Hospital for Sick Children, he asked, "What's the difference between a major and a minor illness?" He waited only a heartbeat before answering, "That all depends on whose kid it is!" A little pediatric humour . . . but he is absolutely right—when it is your own kid, an illness is always major.

Our questions to the Sick Children's medical staff were practical: What should you know as a parent and guardian that will help you help your kids through their journey as patients? How can you ensure that they have the best care available? What tools do you need in your toolbox to navigate the system (especially when you don't live next door to Sick Children's Hospital)? This chapter will answer those questions.

Bringing Baby Home

As you'll recall from Chapter 1, mothers are being discharged from hospital earlier than they were in the past. The average hospital stay for a healthy woman having a rather uncomplicated delivery is about 24 to 48 hours, although it varies across Canada. Twenty years ago, women often stayed in the hospital close to five days for an uncomplicated birth. This trend to shorter lengths of stay is a result of mothers' requests to go home earlier and the need to control hospital costs.

Canadian Institute of Health Information (CIHI) data show that with the decrease in the number of hospital days, there is a higher readmission rate for newborns suffering from jaundice. However, according to the Canadian Paediatric Society (CPS), healthy, full-term babies can be discharged safely from hospital when they are two days old or even earlier so long as they have had a full physical examination and after it is established that the baby has

- a normal temperature,
- had two successful normal feedings,
- urinated,
- had at least one bowel movement,
- received all necessary medications, such as antibiotics to prevent an eye infection, and vitamin K,
- received any necessary immunizations, and
- undergone screening tests to detect certain problems.

The CPS also advises that the mother should have the following supports in place before taking baby home:

- Training for baby care (usually taken in the months before delivery)
- Advice and information on feeding and on detecting health concerns such as jaundice, dehydration, and infection (this is very important since these health issues could be very serious; to understand the signs and symptoms, get a good child-care book and consult the Caring for Kids website—see the Resource Guide at the end of the chapter)

- A health care professional who will provide care for the baby (this is important because there are definitely things that need to be assessed soon after the baby is born—see below)
- A proper car seat
- A list of available community resources or employed support if required to help with routine baby care, breastfeeding, and emergency situations

Prenatal classes are widely available; you can ask your doctor and he or she will be able to direct you. These programs are often run in the hospital in which you will deliver. If you require additional support (such as a doula) or additional navigation, the contact at the hospital will usually be a great resource. Prenatal classes are an excellent way to acquire knowledge and confidence about birthing as well as about the early days of caring for your newborn.

Before you are discharged from the hospital, your baby will be weighed and examined for general health issues, including jaundice and dehydration. At that time, all required screening tests should be completed. Last but not least, the assessment will ensure that breastfeeding is going well and that the family is coping well with the birth of the infant. If you are having your baby at home with the assistance of a certified midwife, you need to ask where these tests will be conducted and how they are to be arranged.

Breastfeeding

If you've ever seen the movie *Blue Lagoon*, starring Brooke Shields, you might have got the idea that breastfeeding is easy. When Brooke tried to feed her newborn the same thing she ate, she was shocked that the baby wouldn't eat it. But one day she lifted baby to her breast and—voilà—baby just latched on. Some women will have an experience this easy, but many will not.

Although breastfeeding is on the rise in Canada, there is not much support that's covered by the health care system. Breastfeeding clinics provide services outside the home. They are typically provided through a hospital, and when they are, they are covered by medicare. You will need to travel to the clinic to get assistance, which is sometimes tough. But they have expert staff to help you as you learn the art. Another resource is a public health nurse; most jurisdictions in Canada have public health nurses. The services differ from province to province. For example, in Ontario the Healthy Babies, Healthy Children program phones all postpartum mothers within a few days of the date of discharge with the offer of a follow-up home visit. Where they consider it beneficial, public health nurses may provide referrals to community services such as breastfeeding, nutrition and health services, play and parenting programs, and child-care services for all families with children up to age six. Not all jurisdictions have such a thorough program, however; the public health department of your province, region, or city is a great place to visit to find what type of breastfeeding supports (and other supports) are offered at the community level.

Francesca found breastfeeding difficult in the beginning—her baby was simply not cooperating! When she needed help at home, she hired a lactation consultant. These consultants are not cheap and may cost over a hundred dollars for a home visit. They will come to your home and watch you breastfeed and suggest changes and offer other advice. Many also offer to sell you equipment such as breast pumps. If you go this route, try to find a certified lactation consultant. Lactation consultants do not need to be certified, but those who are certified receive this designation from the International Board of Certified Lactation Consultants (IBCLC) after they have passed a Board examination. Also, the Board requires the consultant to have completed university- or college-level course work and clinical training. Certification is good for five years, then the consultant must be recertified. You can find a lactation consultant through your hospital by asking the nurse. Your obstetrician, doctor, nurse-practitioner, midwife, or doula may have a listing if these services are available in your area. We agree with those who argue that if the Canadian system provided women with better insured supports, many women would not abandon the breastfeeding experience as quickly as they do. Whether you can or cannot find help that is covered by medicare, it is good to seek out some help if you are struggling. We have included a directory website in the Resource Guide at the end of this chapter.

No matter how hard they try, some women just find it too difficult to continue to breastfeed. Francesca learned that her baby had a severe allergy to milk protein. In her case, it became necessary to stop breastfeeding. While she believed "breast is best," second best was more viable. Some mothers find that they are made to feel inadequate and uncaring if they choose or are forced to stop breastfeeding. Be clear on what you are looking for. If you want to stop breastfeeding because somehow it doesn't seem to be working, there are organizations that can get you back on track—for example, the La Leche League of Canada. However, if you are looking for support in making the transition from breastfeeding to bottle feeding, you don't want to be made to feel guilty.

We do not want to advise on the merits or drawbacks of breastfeeding. It is a debate that is politically charged, and there is sound evidence on both sides of the debate. A good piece of advice is to know where you personally stand on the issue. The question of breastfeeding over bottle feeding is one that's best thought through before you have the baby. Don't forget to consider what your preferred options would be if you couldn't breastfeed. It is crucial to seek out the help of a doctor, midwife, doula, or support organization that fits your belief system. If you hold a moderate view on the subject, make sure that the assistance and advice you get comes from a provider or provider organization with similar views. If you firmly believe in breastfeeding, make sure the people you are going to be relying on are not quick to hand out the "abandon ship" advice. But also make sure that they are knowledgeable, positive, and capable of guiding you and providing you with the support and information you need. It's important you have support that can be available to you either in a clinic or at home, because over-the-phone assistance is often not enough—breastfeeding is pretty much a hands-on affair!

Tips

Do some research and know yourself and your beliefs; decide how important breastfeeding is to you. Seek out the help of someone who shares your belief system.

If you want to breastfeed, make sure the hospital you go to has a good reputation for breastfeeding assistance from the nursing staff and ask them to help you from the start. Push those qualified to help you at the beginning. Bad habits can and do lead to a very painful experience that can prejudice your views about the entire undertaking. If you want to hire someone to help (like a doula or lactation consultant), do so from the start!

Find out by asking your caregiver (doctor, nurse, midwife, or doula) or ask at your hospital if there is a local breastfeeding clinic, covered by your province, that can help with support.

Choosing a Doctor for Your Baby

Should your baby have a pediatrician or a family doctor?

First of all, for most of us, this is a moot point. The fact is that unless you live in a large urban centre, chances are you will not have access to a pediatrician unless your child develops a complex health problem requiring referral by the family doctor. A pediatrician is a medical doctor who has spent an additional four years specializing in the diagnosis and management of childhood diseases. This extra training introduces doctors to specific diseases that are prevalent in children. In addition, they learn how children manifest certain symptoms that may not appear to the same degree or in the same way in adults. Added to the complexity of pediatrics is the challenge that small children do not have the same capacity to express their symptoms, which makes diagnosis a little trickier.

In larger urban centres where health care resources are more plentiful, some pediatricians operate community practices for children. They provide routine services to healthy children and do not require a referral from a family doctor. However, an increasing number of pediatricians have hospital-based practices, and they provide services only to children who require a specialist on a referral basis. Some hospital-based pediatricians also have a community-based practice where they see the more complex cases on a referral basis. Some community pediatricians practise in groups so there is always a doctor on call during daytime hours, even on weekends. If you have the luxury of acquiring access to a pediatrician who practises in this way and is taking on new patients, do it!

Most of us will not have access to a pediatrician to provide the routine care for our child, but we can assure you that if your child is generally healthy, he or she will probably be well served by your family doctor. Family doctors do receive some specialized training in childhood diseases and conditions during their two-year family medicine residency.

The most important point is that whoever provides medical care to your child should be someone who has practical experience (and lots of it). Francesca's father believed that in medicine there is no substitute for experience: The more rashes you see, the easier it becomes to distinguish what you are looking at. The pediatricians we've spoken to maintain that experience is really important in the choice of provider for your child.

The importance of experience is made clear in an Ontario study called "Volume Matters." The study looked at two-year-old children in Ontario to see the relationship between immunization rates and the type of pediatric provider they had. The study conclusions were shocking: Even though all these kids were eligible for free immunizations and they all had free health care, the rate of complete, up-to-date immunization coverage was low (only 66 percent of them had received all the recommended shots by age two). This was despite the fact that on average, these children had 19 visits with providers over the course of a two-year period. On average, the free shots that these kids were eligible to receive at the time the study was conducted would have required no more than five visits to the doctor or nurse-practitioner. Even more surprising, the study showed that children whose providers didn't see a lot of children in their practice were only half as likely to get all the right shots as the children whose providers saw a lot of children in their practice. The study also revealed some other factors associated with kids not being up to date with immunizations: The provider had not been in practice for more than five years (once again, lack of experience) and there was low continuity of care.

Interestingly, the study showed that there was no difference in immunization coverage for children receiving care from family doctors compared to those receiving care from pediatricians—a testament to our belief that for regular pediatric care, your child is fine with a family doctor, provided the doctor sees a lot of children.

Tip

Choose a doctor for your child who looks after a lot of other children.

Although this study looked only at immunization rates, the principle is the same; more experience results in more efficient and effective care.

To help you choose the right doctor for your child, here are some questions you should ask:

1. Does this doctor see a lot of kids? How do you know? Take a look around the office. Are there kids in the waiting room? Are there toys or children's books? Are the patients you typically see in the waiting room elderly or do many of them look like they could have kids themselves? Just by looking around, you can tell something about the kind of age group the doctor treats. You may also consider asking the doctor if he or she treats many infants and children. It is more important that the doctor has a practice in which he or she sees a large number of children than it is for you to have the same doctor as your child.
2. Does this doctor care about kids? How does he or she relate to the child? Does the doctor seem to like children? This may all seem very touchy-feely, but with kids, part of the battle is getting the child to feel comfortable with the doctor. As your children grow up, this becomes very important, especially when they need to discuss difficult topics like sexuality.
3. How available is your doctor? Will he or she fit your child in on an emergency basis if your child is sick and needs to be seen? This is very important for anyone, but especially so for infants and small children. If you think you'll need to wait a week for an appointment, you need a backup plan such as going to your hospital's emergency department

or going to a different doctor. Sometimes waiting for an appointment is all right, but with childhood illness, at times it is not.

> **Tip**
>
> Phone the doctor after hours or on the weekend and find out what the answering machine says. If it directs you to leave a message (because the messages are monitored), that is a good sign. If it provides a number to call or another physician on call, that is also good. What is less good is a message directing you to go to the nearest overcrowded emergency department, which means that the doctor provides no after-hours support.
>
> If you live in an urban centre, it helps to have a doctor who is on staff at a local hospital.

What You Can Do to Ensure Better Care

The first step in ensuring excellent care for your child involves understanding that children need to be followed more closely than adults. One of the defining features of sickness in children is that it can progress more rapidly than in adults. Dr. Marvin Gans explains that a child can have a cold at noon and develop a dangerously high fever with a bad bacterial infection within a few hours.

Frequently, parents will take their child to the doctor, who will conclude that the child has a viral infection. But, with kids, that diagnosis may change quickly. And when the child starts running a very high fever, the parents often feel too intimidated and reluctant to march right back to the doctor, having seen her only three hours earlier. The thinking is that if doc said at noon that Johnny was going to be okay, then what more is there to add at 3:00 P.M.? But with kids, things can change fast. Be prepared for this. And be prepared to act.

Another common misperception that occurs when we bring our children to a doctor or nurse-practitioner is that there is always an answer—a clear diagnosis with a clear treatment. Instead, with kids many things develop with time. It is often the case that the provider will tell you that he or she is not certain what is going on. That is normal. The important thing, then, is that you don't leave the office without a list of what you should look for over the next hours or days (don't forget your paper and pencil when you leave home!).

Tip

Ask the doctor or nurse-practitioner what you should be looking for and what should or should not happen next.

What would be a worrisome sign that indicates you should bring the child back?

Kids can get better very quickly. But they also tend to get sick and deteriorate very quickly. This simple fact has some important repercussions for you as a parent or guardian. Dr. Gans and Dr. Jeremy Friedman, head of pediatric medicine at the Hospital for Sick Children, shared some tips:

1. Don't be shy about taking your little one right back to the doctor if you feel that his or her condition has changed for the worse. People tend not to appreciate that illness progresses. A diagnosis may not be apparent early on and the child can also deteriorate rapidly (as children often do). Nip the problem in the bud and don't let it fester. Dithering and waiting around is worse for the child, worse for you, and worse for the health care system.
2. Continuity of care makes establishing a diagnosis easier. If your child was seen by a particular doctor and seems to be worse, take him or her back to the same doctor. If your child was seen in the emergency department, take him or her back to the same emergency department. Dr. Gans explains that this is sometimes counterintuitive to many parents. You bring the child to the emergency department and they don't make her better. You bring her home and she gets worse. The parent might assume that the hospital didn't provide quality care, so they take the child elsewhere. But a diagnosis is like putting a puzzle together. Pieces of information that were gathered at the first medical visit may provide tremendous insight on the second visit. By taking the child back to the same place, you allow the doctor to have access to this information. Here is an example that Dr. Gans provides:

A child with bad vomiting and diarrhea is seen in the emergency department at 9:00 A.M. He is checked, weighed, and sent home. That night, the child is worse. The parent takes the child back to the same hospital emergency department. The doctor on call finds the information from the child's last visit and notices that the child's weight was 33 pounds (15 kg). The doctor weighs the child this time and now he is only 28 pounds (13 kg). The child is treated for dehydration. It would have taken a lot longer to establish that the child was dehydrated if the second doctor didn't have access to the child's weight from that morning.

3. When it comes to diagnosis, history can be very important. Be prepared to communicate your child's history, even if you are not asked. At times we may be forced into circumstances where we can't take our children to the same doctor or medical centre. Once when Francesca was travelling, her daughter was complaining about a sore ear. At a walk-in clinic, the doctor checked her ears. He said one was a little red but he was not inclined to prescribe antibiotics for that. Because Francesca knows that ear irritations in kids can turn into nasty bacterial infections quickly, she told the doctor her daughter's history—how she had suffered many ear infections and how she actually ruptured the membrane in her ear once due to a bad infection. The doctor immediately changed his

mind. He wrote out a prescription saying that with that kind of history, he did not want to take any chances. Francesca was not trying to coerce the doctor into writing a prescription, but she was providing as much information as she could. If a doctor has never seen your child before, chances are he or she has no information. You can be a tremendous help by supplying your child's medical history. Knowing their allergies is also essential.

4. If you go to the emergency department or to a walk-in clinic, don't leave without making a note of any tests done, what was checked (your child's weight, for example), and any test results provided. Ask for a photocopy of the test results. People often think that the health care system is one big seamless, well-organized system. Maybe it should be, but it isn't. If you visit the emergency department with your child, and you have given them the name of your family doctor, you probably think that your doctor will be notified immediately of any test results and given a summary report of the child's visit. While that should be the case, it ain't necessarily so. It will take your doctor many times longer to procure this information after the fact than it will take you to get a photocopy on the spot. Dr. Friedman also points out that while the hospital health team usually records the findings of emergency visits in duplicate so they can send one part to your family doctor, often the address is

wrong or illegible. At times the copy doesn't arrive at your child's practitioner at all. Other times, phone calls are received by an answering machine and the phone tag between your child's doctor and the hospital begins. So make sure you leave the emergency department or walk-in clinic with a list of what was checked, tests that were taken, and results that were received.

5. Tell the doctor why you are taking notes. It is interesting to talk to a doctor about the idea of taking notes. You will discover that this is a major theme of this book, yet we had never considered the doctor's interpretation of the patient's taking notes. Since we have interviewed several physicians, we now know it is good practice to explain to the doctor up front why you are doing this! The doctor may think that you are creating a record in case he or she messes up. Explain clearly that you may need to go somewhere else and it may be helpful to have a record of what this visit yields.
6. Go with your gut! Trust your instincts and be the squeaky wheel if you sense something is really wrong with your child. Both Dr. Friedman and Dr. Gans agree with this. At the medical school where Dr. Gans teaches, he tells his interns that they ignore parental (especially maternal) instinct at their little patient's peril. A common theme of hospital horror stories about children being released only to die soon after is that the

parent or guardian sensed there was something horribly amiss with the child but erred on the side of deference toward the doctor or medical centre. It's all too easy to think, "After all, I am not a doctor. The doctor must be right and I must be wrong." If you aren't satisfied and you really feel something is very wrong, here are some things you should do:

- Ask your doctor to refer you to a pediatrician.
- Take the child to a university hospital, a children's hospital, or a regional centre *where there are pediatricians*.
- Discuss clearly why you are concerned and what has been done to date for your child (tests or treatment).
- If your child has been seen repeatedly for a problem with no resolution or diagnosis, tell the pediatrician: "Doctor, you are the third (second, fourth, *whatever)* physician to see my child, and here are the tests that have been done to date and the results."

7. During a hospital stay, be involved in your child's care in a positive way. Don't make enemies with the staff. If they seem abrupt, it's likely overwork, not malice. Try to work with them positively. People who are treated with respect and a smile tend to respond in kind. Confrontations are not generally productive (though at times they are needed and later in the book we discuss tactics—

see Chapter 14, "Be the Squeaky Wheel"). But before you start sounding off, try some of these techniques first:

- Enlist the staff's help.
- Explain why you are worried. Share your fears. People—especially people who work in hospitals—generally like to help people who are afraid.
- Talk to the right person—if it is a medical problem, talk to the doctor taking care of your child. If you are having trouble communicating with the doctor, the nursing staff may be able to run some interference for you, and the doctor may help run interference with the nursing staff as well.

8. Always carry your child's health insurance card and immunization record with you when making visits to a care provider. If you are going to the hospital for tests or treatment, bring the plastic hospital card as well. These are essential to receiving timely, hassle-free, informed care.
9. Be an advocate for your child and persevere! Dr. Friedman says that while everyone should have an advocate in the hospital, little children need an advocate even more than adults. Dr. Friedman is always worried when he enters a child's room in the hospital and sees no adult there. Be an advocate outside of the hospital too. You know your child better than anyone, and that is

why your child needs you. Be vocal and persistent in a calm, constructive way.

10. Get a good reference book or reference information on child care! You must have a good book that talks about diseases that affect children. By good, we mean reputable and credible. The book should describe signs and symptoms, discuss treatments and general pediatric care, and explain what needs to happen when. Several great books are listed in the Resource Guide at the end of this chapter.
    Dr. Friedman is very concerned about the number of parents who rely on less than credible Internet sites. There is nothing wrong with the Internet, except that its ability to deliver good advice is dependent on the credibility of the website. Make sure you are visiting sites that have been recommended by your doctor or nurse. Visit sites created by teaching hospitals, universities, national agencies, doctors, or nurses—in short, sites with peer review to ensure accurate information.

Immunization

Infectious diseases used to be the number-one killer worldwide and now account for under 5 percent of deaths in Canada. The Canadian Paediatric Society reports that this is largely owing to immunization programs, which have saved more lives in Canada over the last 50 years than any other health intervention.

You may be surprised to know that not all the important vaccines your child should have are covered by medicare. Coverage (as with other items) is dependent on where you live. For example, at one time Ontario did not cover the costs of chickenpox, pneumococcal, and meningococcal vaccines. However, these vaccines are now fully covered in Ontario. Though these vaccines are costly, it is important that your child receive them whether or not they are covered in your province or territory.

One big mistake that a parent might make is to assume that the doctor or nurse-practitioner will monitor his child's vaccinations perfectly. Many do. Some don't. And, as shown above, different caregivers often do not share records that indicate what your child has received and when his or her next immunization is due.

Michael Decter tells of a small community that has worked to rectify this problem. In September 2005 he was visiting Haines Junction, Yukon Territory. It's in a beautiful setting at the foot of Mount Logan on the edge of Kluane National Park. Michael was part of an outreach effort of the Health Council of Canada. The nurses gave them a tour of the Haines Nursing station. From this two-storey building four nurses, two full-time and two part time, look after the primary-care needs of 800 residents in Haines Junction and the surrounding area. Many aspects, from telemedicine to the diagnostic capability, were innovative and impressive. The most interesting aspect was the immunization record. Building from a simple software program provided by

Health Canada, the nurses had created their own electronic health record. For each of the children in the community, the record posted immunization notices so they could be scheduled for their routine vaccines. In one of the most remote corners of Canada a nurse-led primary-care approach was doing a terrific job on immunizations. Many busy urban physicians do not have as organized and systematic a process for ensuring that their young patients receive all vaccines and booster shots on schedule.

There are only three fundamental rules regarding vaccinations:

1. Make certain your child receives all the vaccines that are recommended by the Canadian Paediatric Society, regardless of whether they are covered in your jurisdiction.
2. Make certain that you bring your child in for his or her vaccination at the right time for that particular vaccine. This is very important in order for the vaccine to be effective in protecting your child. Ask for a record book to keep track and bring it with you to all your child's visits.
3. Know that the schedule of when your child should be vaccinated may differ a little from province to province, so make sure to talk to your doctor if you are moving, to ensure that your child doesn't miss a vaccination.

If you aren't certain what the recommended vaccines are, here is what's recommended by the Canadian Paediatric Society and Health Canada's National Advisory Committee on Immunization:

- 5-in-1 vaccine (also known as DPTP-Hib): protects against diphtheria, pertussis (whooping cough), tetanus, polio, and *Haemophilus influenzae* type b (Hib). *Haemophilus influenzae* type b is a bacteria that can infect the fluid around the brain and spinal cord. Hib can cause meningitis as well as other serious diseases that can result in brain damage or death. In Canada, most infants get this shot at 2, 4, 6, and 18 months of age.
- 4-in-1 vaccine: protects against diphtheria, tetanus, pertussis, and polio. In Canada children get this shot at four to six years of age.
- MMR vaccine: protects against measles, mumps, and rubella. Two doses are required, the first at 12 months and the second at either 18 months or before the child begins school. This vaccine is covered in all provinces and territories.
- Hepatitis B vaccine: protects against hepatitis B and is given either in infancy or between the ages of 9 and 13.
- dTap vaccine: vaccine for adolescents that protects against diphtheria, tetanus, and pertussis.
- Chickenpox vaccine: protects against this common childhood illness. It is given generally at 12 months.

- Pneumococcal vaccine: protects against infections caused by *Streptococcus pneumoniae*, including meningitis (a brain infection), pneumonia, and ear infections. It is given at 2, 4, 6, and 12 months.
- Meningococcal vaccine: protects against diseases caused by the *Meningococcus* bacteria, including meningitis and septicemia, a serious blood infection. It is given at 12 months.
- Acellular pertussis vaccine: has recently been added to the Canadian vaccine schedule, though it is not covered by all provincial and territorial health plans. The sixth dose of pertussis vaccine, given at around 15 years of age, will help prevent teenagers from getting pertussis, which in adolescents can range from a prolonged cough to a severe illness. The Canadian Paediatric Society recommends that all provinces implement programs to give an adolescent booster dose of acellular pertussis vaccine.

The first five vaccines are usually covered by your provincial or territorial health plan. The last four vaccines are not always covered but are considered very important. A chart that shows which jurisdictions cover these four vaccines and which do not can be found at www.caringforkids.ca—click on the Immunization link.

Your doctor can advise you on

- which vaccines are covered in your jurisdiction;
- whether a flu shot is right for your child;

- which vaccine(s) your child will need if you are travelling;
- what to do if your child has any type of reaction after getting a vaccination;
- what to give your child to avoid fever or pain after a vaccine.

Most provinces and territories offer vaccine programs for high-risk children. Consult your doctor, public health nurse, or public health office for details. If your child is very sick when it's time for a vaccine, talk to your doctor. If your child has a cold and no fever, he or she should still be able to receive the vaccination.

Your Adolescent Child

So far we have discussed navigating care only for infants and very young children, with the exception of the one vaccine aimed at adolescents, acellular pertussis. This is largely because more medical intervention is required when children are small.

Choosing a doctor for your teen involves different criteria than choosing one for an infant or younger child. Generally, because many of the health issues affecting teens can be driven by complex issues such as sexual concerns, peer pressure, low self-esteem, or possibly other mental health issues, it is important at this age more than any other that your child have a trusting relationship with his or her doctor. This can mean that the child may not be comfortable visiting the same doctor you visit. He or she may not want to confide in your doctor about concerns, questions, or problems if it appears that the doctor will disclose his or her secrets to you on your next visit. At times it may be best to steer your teen to a different doctor from your own.

There are a number of serious issues that tend to affect adolescents. Unfortunately, while many of these issues are either caused by health problems or have significant health implications, there are not many supports in Canada to deal with them. This is particularly true in the case of some mental health problems that can lead to substance abuse, eating disorders, or even suicide. Here parents must be vigilant, observant, and creative to find supports and work to solve or control these problems. Obesity is a concern attracting more attention and is another problem that can severely affect the health of a child, teen, and later adult. These next sections will look at some of these issues.

Mental Health Problems in Kids

It is clear that there are some major problems affecting young people in Canada, and that these problems are rooted in mental health. Teenagers and young adults are more likely than people in any other age group to have mental health disorders, yet they are the least likely to seek help in dealing with their problems. The sad truth is that mental health problems are often difficult to diagnose. They can range from schizophrenia to eating disorders, from depression to alcoholism. Sometimes symptoms are sporadic. Other times (as in the case with some eating disorders) they can be hidden by the young person. Parents should consult reputable books on mental health issues, especially those listed at the end of this chapter, to find out about the possible warning signs. Clearly, a professional assessment will help.

According to an article in the *Canadian Journal of Psychiatry* published in 2002, of the approximately 7.5 million children living in Canada, a little over 1 million under the age of 15 have mental health problems. These conditions affect their lives at home and at school, and many of these disorders will carry on into adulthood. The rates of mental health problems are higher after the age of 15. Mental health issues can range from attention deficit disorder in the early years to concerns about low self-esteem, eating disorders, and beyond in later years. In adolescence, low self-esteem appears to be of particular concern: In 2002, Health Canada reported that 25 percent of boys and 36 percent of girls in Grade 10 experienced feeling low, and the Public Health Agency of Canada reports that hospitalization for eating disorders in 15-year-old girls increased by 34 percent between 1987 and 1999.

According to CIHI statistics, alcohol use reported by Canadian adolescents has risen remarkably. In its *Report on Mental Illnesses in Canada*, Health Canada shows that heavy drinking is increasing in all age groups—particularly adolescent males. Statistics Canada reports that about one-third of youths between the ages of 12 and 17

Prevalence of Mental Disorders in Canadian Children

	Estimated Prevalence (%)	Approximate Number in Canada
Any anxiety disorder	6.4	507,000
Attention-deficit hyperactivity disorder	4.8	380,000
Conduct disorder	4.2	333,000
Any depressive disorder	3.5	277,000
Substance abuse	0.8	63,000
Pervasive developmental disorder	0.3	24,000
Obsessive-compulsive disorder	0.2	16,000
Any eating disorder	0.1	8,000
Tourette's syndrome	0.1	8,000
Schizophrenia	0.1	8,000
Bipolar disorder	< 0.1	<8,000
Any disorder	14.3	1,134,000

Source: Health Council of Canada, "Their Future Is Now: Healthy Choices for Canada's Children," 2006.

reported using marijuana in 2001, and 13 percent of youths in the same age group reported using illicit drugs such as cocaine or crack. Almost 3 out of every 100 adolescents in that age group are dependent on drugs.

Suicide is another serious concern for young Canadians and particularly Aboriginal youths, for whom the rates tend to be about three to six times the national average. Although Statistics Canada reports that suicide rates for youths dropped a little between 2000 and 2003, suicide still accounts for 9 percent of deaths in 10- to 14-year-olds, and 22 percent of deaths in 15- to 19-year-olds. We don't know the number of youths attempting suicide.

Another often overlooked problem for adolescents is homelessness. It is difficult to ascertain how many teens are homeless. CIHI cites research showing it tends to be more prevalent among young males than females and it is also prevalent in Aboriginal youths. It also reports that homeless youths are at a higher risk for injuries, poor health, violence, sexually transmitted diseases, suicide, other mental health issues, and a whole host of other concerns.

What You Can Do

It is hard to do anything to help your child if you don't suspect a problem. A good relationship between you and your child can be very important in noticing symptoms and in making your child feel comfortable enough with you to let you into his or her world and speak to you about issues that might be of concern. Fostering a good relationship with your child is always important regardless of what stage of life he or she is in, of course. However, when it comes to adolescent mental health issues, a good relationship can be the difference between suspecting something is up or not. Though even the best relationship does not necessarily mean that a parent or guardian will notice a problem, it can help. Try to get to know who your children are hanging out with and what they are doing. Involve yourself in their lives. This can be tough because young people at this age tend to want to assert their independence. There are professionals who can give advice on how to accomplish this balancing act, including psychologists and counsellors. Some religious organizations provide counselling services in their community. Ask your doctor. Visit your jurisdiction's website for listings of community services in this area.

Just as you were an advocate for your young child, you also need to be an advocate for your older children when mental health disorders are suspected, Dr. Friedman maintains. Hospitals often have assessment services, but unfortunately, they often do not have many services set up to deal with these potentially serious issues. Your family doctor is usually a good person to help you navigate and can arrange an assessment in a hospital or with a mental health professional. Some family doctors do provide counselling services; however, if the issue is serious, they will probably refer your child to a specialist for assessment.

Community health agencies have mental health services, but there is a great deal of inconsistency in the level of help you can get from one community to another. Also wait times for community services are often very long. There are charitable organizations and associations that are dedicated to different mental health issues. These organizations sometimes have programs to help youths overcome mental health problems or they can provide navigational support to those who can. In the Resource Guide, we list a few of these organizations.

> **Tip**
>
> Take any sign of mental illness as seriously as you do a physical ailment. Seek help for your child.

Obesity in Children

Francesca's work colleague once told her, "I have tried everything to lose weight." Then she added, "Except diet and exercise." When it comes to childhood obesity, there is a great deal of truth in this statement.

For most of us, diet and exercise are the magic combination for weight control. That isn't different when it comes to children. When Francesca became a parent, she discovered how easy it can be to let kids develop bad eating habits without meaning to or even realizing it. Her daughter quickly caught on to her weakness for peace and quiet, and it wasn't long before Smarties, fizzy pop, chips, and the like became staples on the grocery list as rewards for not hassling Mum. After about a month of outright lunacy, Francesca changed her ways—and her daughter's eating habits.

Children sometimes go through a period when their appetite isn't terribly good. They may be healthy, happy, and active, but they just don't seem to want to eat much. We assuage our worry by tempting our child to eat things we normally wouldn't allow on the dinner table—junk food, in other words. We should remember what the sensible Dr. Gans told Francesca: Small children don't usually starve themselves. If they are happy and active and have no illness, forcing them isn't the way to go.

Unhealthy eating and lack of physical activity are contributing to childhood obesity. Although obesity may have stabilized in recent years, more than 1 million Canadian children are overweight and half a million are obese. Overweight kids are often unhappy kids—children can be cruel to one another, and overweight kids generally get a rough ride from their peers. Also, they often grow up to be overweight adults. Obesity can lead to serious health problems in the future, including type 2 diabetes, sleep apnea, and high cholesterol. Many of these problems promote heart attacks and other life-threatening conditions.

Here are some facts to consider if you're worried about your child's weight:

- Children between the ages of 6 and 11 who spend more than two hours in front of television and computer screens are twice as likely to be overweight as those who logged one hour or less per day.
- Half of Canada's children and young people watch between two and four hours of television each day.
- The amount of time that Canadian children spend in front of computers is among the highest in the world.

- According to a survey conducted by the World Health Organization, fewer than half the youths in Canada under 16 reported eating fruits and vegetables more than once per day despite the recommendations in the *Canada Food Guide* of between 5 and 10 servings.
- Active Healthy Kids Canada reported Statistics Canada data showing that fewer than half of Canadian children and youths are active enough each day to meet the Health Canada guidelines for healthy growth and development.
- A link between body weight and socio-economic status has been documented in an articled published in the *Canadian Journal of Public Health*. Children who live in neighbourhoods with higher unemployment rates, lower average family incomes, or fewer neighbours with post-secondary education are at greater risk of being overweight or obese than children in higher-income neighbourhoods. These children are also less likely to participate in organized physical activities.
- Statistics Canada reports that obesity rates differ from jurisdiction to jurisdiction and tend to be higher in eastern Canada.

What You Can Do

First off, be honest with yourself about the status of your child's weight. If your child is obviously overweight, stop the excuses. Stop telling yourself, "He'll grow out of it."

He might. Then again he might not. Often, a child with bad eating habits will lose a lot of weight when his metabolism increases in his teens, but frequently, if the bad habits don't change, he will gain the weight again when he is older. Bottom line: You can't take chances. Deal with it now. Eating habits need to be corrected early.

Get a good book or seek the help of a professional (certified dietitian, nutritionist, nurse, or doctor) if your child requires a change in diet. Obviously, if your child eats nothing but high-calorie junk food and sits in front of the television all day, you probably do not need a professional to tell you that isn't good. However, you may need some help replacing sweet or salty snacks or high-calorie foods to ensure that your child's diet is balanced. *The Canada Food Guide* (*Canada's Guide to Healthy Eating and Physical Activity* at www.hc-sc.gc.ca) offers a great deal of help in this area.

Don't "kill" your kid with love. Often parents mean well and may be overfeeding their little ones out of a misplaced sense of love to express their caring.

Make sure your kid is active. Operating the remote control quickly does not constitute activity. If your child is on the computer for two hours a night, it may be too much, especially if he or she is not doing any other physical activities.

Most important, you are your children's key role model. If you want them to be physically active, then put on your walking shoes or dust the cobwebs off your bike and get out with them! If you collapse in front of the TV with a big bag of chips and a can of pop, do you honestly expect your children not to want to do the same?

Dr. Gans observes that in large urban centres especially, there seems to be a shortage of spontaneous activity. That is to say, most basketball courts are empty, and kids don't play road hockey on their own. It seems we are in a society where all activity needs to be organized. Kids need to be "enrolled" in programs. Why not try to get a game of road hockey going on your street? Take your kids skating. Get them involved in a snowball fight in the yard. Or try to organize some kind of inclusive activity in your neighbourhood.

Tip

To develop healthy eating and exercise habits, your children need to have your behaviour as an example.

RESOURCE GUIDE

BOOKS

Caring for Kids: The Complete Canadian Guide to Children's Health. Norman Saunders and Jeremy Friedman (Toronto: Key Porter Books, 2006).

This book is a comprehensive contemporary guide to health and wellness in children up to the age of 10. It combines medically sound care with cutting-edge research. With information taken from the best scientific evidence available, the authors provide a thoughtful, compassionate, and informed approach to an extensive array of childhood conditions and illnesses. It is written by world-renowned providers of children's health care and published in cooperation with Toronto's Hospital for Sick Children.

The book is divided into three main sections. The first part deals with some of the more important symptoms that parents must identify and manage. In the second part, parents will find information on the nature of many specific conditions that affect children. This section seeks to answer three key questions: What is the condition? What can parents expect to happen? How should the problem be treated? The third part of this guide is a reference section to help manage some of the common accidents and emergencies that occur in childhood.

Your Child's Best Shot: A Parent's Guide to Vaccination. Ronald Gold (Ottawa: Canadian Paediatric Society, 2002).

This book answers questions such as

- Does my child need all these shots?
- Do vaccines really work?
- Are the vaccines safe?

First published by the Canadian Paediatric Society in 1997, *Your Child's Best Shot* is a definitive source of information on vaccines and immunization programs for parents nationwide.

Dr. Jack Newman's Guide to Breastfeeding. Jack Newman and Teresa Pitman (Toronto: HarperCollins, 2000).

Newman, a Canadian pediatrician, writing with Teresa Pitman, offers up-to-date advice on all aspects of breastfeeding: getting off to the best start, preventing and dealing with common problems, breastfeeding premature babies and babies with special needs, and breastfeeding during illness or separation. This book is for health professionals and breastfeeding women.

ORGANIZATIONS AND ASSOCIATIONS

Canadian Paediatric Society
www.cps.ca
www.caringforkids.cps.ca
These two websites are interrelated. The Canadian Paediatric Society (CPS) website offers services to parents and caregivers by routing them to the second website, called "Caring for Kids," which has been developed by the CPS. Caring for Kids is extremely helpful for accessing information on health and wellness issues, including behavioural problems, immunizations, what to do when your child is ill, and many others. You can also look for a local doctor who has a children's practice if you click on "Find a Doctor" and a local children's

hospital if you click on "Find a Hospital." The Canadian Paediatric Society also has a great on-line bookstore.

Canadian Coalition for Immunization Awareness and Promotion
www.immunize.cpha.ca
This site has information for parents, children, and health professionals on immunizations.

Breastfeeding.com
www.breastfeeding.com
This international website can help you locate a lactation consultant in your province or territory. It is tricky to navigate to the Canadian directory link, so here it is: www.breastfeeding.com/directory/states/canada.html.

La Leche League of Canada
www.llli.org (international)
www.allaitement.ca (French Canada)
www.llli.ca (English Canada)
Telephone: 1-800-665-4324
This organization is a very strong supporter of breastfeeding. It provides breastfeeding education and support to mothers in Canada. Through the website, you can access breastfeeding help near you, ask questions, and join support groups.

Sheena's Place
www.sheenasplace.org
This organization provides support for all people with eating disorders, including support for parents and teens. Sheena's Place has developed programs for families, peers, educators, and other care providers at no cost to users. It enlists professionals on a fee-for-service basis, and they provide group support to those identified as having eating disorders and their families. It offers outreach programs to schools, colleges, and universities. You can get a terrific listing of books that parents and teens can read on the subject by visiting the website and clicking on "Library."

GOVERNMENT PROGRAMS

The following information will help you access all the provincial or territorial benefit programs potentially available to your child.

Government of Canada: Canada Benefits
www.canadabenefits.gc.ca
This is an excellent website. To navigate, access the website homepage. Under the first column, labelled "I am" (a parent, a senior, a student), indicate that you are "a parent." Under the second column, called "Life Events," click on "Health Concerns."

Choose your province or territory.

Then choose the area of interest:

- Health and Dental Care (including things like programs that cover assistive devices for children with severe disabilities)
- Mental Health, Counselling, and Addictions
- Prescription Drug Coverage

Children's Mental Health Ontario
www.kidsmentalhealth.ca
Don't worry if you are not from Ontario! If you click on "Links," you will get an excellent list of credible mental health websites that you will be able to link to.

For children's programs, including mental health programs, immunization programs, drug programs for children, and social services available to children in your jurisdiction, contact your province or territory. See the back of the book for these websites and contact numbers. They will usually link you to community services in your region or area.

THREE

Child Safety in Canada

Shortly after Francesca brought her beautiful baby daughter home from the hospital, her sister, Sylvia, gave her some advice: "Your job for the first two years is keepin' 'em alive."

This advice turned out to be quite good. The fact is that the best way to navigate the health care system is to avoid having to access it in the first place. And when it comes to infants and young children, navigation begins with knowing what is and isn't a threat to your child. A great deal of information is available, from a variety of sources. This chapter seeks to bring the most relevant and up-to-date information on the issue of child safety and offers a quick reference on rules and recommendations for helping to keep your child out of the health care system.

The ease with which infants and toddlers locate the most dangerous items and situations is mind-boggling. It is as if they are born with an internal radar device that seeks out brave new hazardous worlds so they can boldly go where no one should go (until he or she is at least 15).

Fortunately for parents, there's an organization called Safe Kids Canada that raises awareness about dangers in the environment your children live in and the products they use. It advocates for safer environments to reduce injury. The organization aims to influence policy-makers and to ensure that the public is aware of what they can do to promote safety. Most of the information in this chapter is based on Safe Kids Canada's reports, information, and educational materials.

In Canada, the single leading cause of death after the first year of life is unintentional injury. And though death rates owing to injury dropped by 37 percent

Main Causes of Unintentional Injury Leading to Death between 1994 and 2003 in Canadian Children

Under 1	1–4 Years	5–9 Years	10–14 Years
Threats to breathing 41%	Drowning 23%	Motor vehicle passenger injury 18%	Motor vehicle passenger injury 19%
Motor vehicle passenger injury 14%	Motor vehicle passenger injury 14%	Pedestrian injury 18%	Pedestrian injury 14%
Drowning 8%	Burns 14%	Drowning 13%	Drowning 10%
	Pedestrian injury 14%	Burns 12%	

Source: Safe Kids Canada. *Child and Youth Unintentional Injury: 10 Years in Review*. Toronto: Safe Kids Canada, 2006.

between 1994 and 2003, it is estimated that about 390 kids under the age of 14 die each year in this country from unintentional injury. Consider, too, that each year an estimated 25,000 kids are hospitalized for the treatment of injuries.

Let's begin with some information about the main causes of unintentional death in children as they are identified in the chart above.

Threats to Breathing

Threats to breathing include choking, suffocation, and strangulation. Deaths caused by threats to breathing tend to be higher in small children, who are more likely to choke on food or small objects and are less able to free themselves from things like bedding. Although deaths caused by threats to breathing seem to be decreasing according to the latest data from the Canadian Institute of Health Information (CIHI) and Statistics Canada, these threats are still the third leading cause of death to Canadian children. By far the greatest threat to breathing is choking, which accounts for as much as 94 percent of all hospitalizations.

Here are some recommendations from Safe Kids Canada to prevent choking:

- Keep nuts, carrots, popcorn, and hard fruits and vegetables away from children under four.
- Keep toys with small parts, coins, batteries, and other such items away from kids under four.

- Do not let children walk about or play while eating. At mealtimes or snack times, kids should be seated with their feet under the table. Dr. Gans mentions that he frequently sees choking problems that have been caused by children who are eating while walking about or not seated properly at a table.

Here are a few things that you can do to avoid suffocation:

- Make certain that cribs don't contain soft mobile bedding such as comforters, pillows, crib bumpers, and stuffed animals when the baby is very small. These items could suffocate a young baby.
- Ensure that the crib is not older than 1986 (check the label) and that the mattress supports are secure enough to prevent the bottom coming loose and the child becoming trapped.

The Canadian Paediatric Society recommends that babies sleep in their own cribs for the first year of their life and not share an adult's bed.

Here are a few things you can do to avoid strangulation:

- Keep curtain and blind cords out of your child's reach.
- Make certain drawstrings on clothing are cut off or well tied.

Motor Vehicle Passenger Injuries

Information from CIHI and Statistics Canada would indicate that generally there has been a slow and steady decrease in deaths and hospitalizations of Canadian children (from newborns to 14-year-olds) who were occupants in motor vehicles. However, as you saw in the chart on page 85, it still remains one of the leading causes of death for kids of all ages.

Research also conclusively tells us that the risk of death is significantly reduced when car seats and booster seats are used and used properly. One study conducted by the Task Force on Community Preventative Services and published in 2001 in the *American Journal of Preventative Medicine* claims that when used correctly, car seats reduce the risk of death by 71 percent for infants under the age of one. Sadly, Safe Kids Canada reports that an estimated 44 to 81 percent of car and booster seats are not used correctly, putting children at risk. Safe Kids Canada also reports in a 2003 survey that nearly three-quarters of Canadian children between the ages of four and nine are not protected by booster seats. Transport Canada recorded in 2005 that 92 percent of infants who sustained severe injuries as passengers were not using the appropriate restraint at the time of the crash. That percentage doesn't go down much for toddlers and it goes up for school-aged kids.

So what is wrong? How is it that in the face of such compelling evidence, our kids are still not being buckled up properly? One problem is that many of us don't know the difference between a booster seat and a car seat and under what circumstances each should be used.

Tip

To find out what regulations are in place for car seats and booster seats in your jurisdiction, call your Ministry of Transportation.

Safe Kids Canada has helped clear up some of the confusion by providing the following information: A car seat uses the seat-belt system in a car to attach the seat to the vehicle. However, it also uses a harness system over the child's bones to protect them in a crash. The harness acts as the seat belt for your child. The harness—a five-point harness is best—places the pressure of a crash or sudden stop over five points on the child's body, whereas a seat belt (shoulder and lap belt) would cross on only three points. Also, an adult seat belt does not fit an infant, toddler, or young child properly, so a car or booster seat is needed. Race car drivers use five-point harness systems—the more points of contact with the body, the less damage will be done in an accident. Car seats are installed facing either the back of the car or the front of the car, depending on the height, weight, and age of the child.

A booster seat is designed as a seat-belt-positioning device for older children who have stronger bone structure and muscles and who have outgrown car seats with a harness system. In this case, the booster seat is not actually attached to the car. The booster seat lifts the child up so that the adult lap and shoulder belts cross the body over hard bone structures—chest bone and hip bones—to absorb crash forces. A child must be big enough for the seat belt to be positioned properly in a booster seat. It is easy to see why moving to a booster seat set-up too soon can be dangerous.

Many forward-facing car seats meant for toddlers and young children can also be used as a booster seat. They come with a harness the child can use until he or she reaches a given height or weight limit, and then can be used as a booster seat without the harness when the child is big enough.

Each province and territory has its own laws regarding the use of car seats and booster seats. These laws use criteria such as age, weight, and height of the child as a guide for which type of seat should be used. Booster seat legislation does not exist in every jurisdiction in the country, however. Only Quebec, Ontario, and Nova Scotia have created legislation for booster seats, with requirements based on age, height, and weight.

Here is what is recommended by Safe Kids Canada:

- Use a rear-facing car seat until the child is at least one year and at least 20 pounds.
- Use a forward-facing car seat until the child is at least 40 pounds (18 kg), which usually occurs between four and five years of age.

- Use a booster seat until the child fits the seat belt correctly, which usually occurs at 57 inches (145 cm) tall and around 80 pounds (36 kg, usually not reached until age nine).

Note that your province or territory's legislations may be different but this is the recommendation.

Safe Kids Canada estimates that 44 to 81 percent of car seats and booster seats are not used correctly. And most kids in Canada between the ages of four and nine do not use booster seats at all. Perhaps the most shocking statistics are these: 92 percent of infants, 74 percent of toddlers, and 96 percent of school-aged kids injured in vehicle crashes were not wearing appropriate restraints at the time.

Here is a list of things you can do to make sure your child is safe on every ride:

- Make certain you have the instructions and all the parts that came with a second-hand car seat. No instructions? Missing parts? Don't use it.
- Make sure whatever car seat or booster seat you buy has a label that says it meets Canadian Motor Vehicle Safety Standards.
- Don't use a car seat or booster seat that is over 10 years old because the plastic parts wear down. Also, check labels and manuals because sometimes the manufacturer puts an expiry date on the product that is less than 10 years.

- Use the right product for your child's weight, height, and age.
- Make sure the harness straps of the car seat or booster seat are snug and not left slack.
- Be sure to install the seat in the vehicle according to the manufacturer's instructions (especially in older vehicles where there isn't a special latch for the car seat or booster seat to hook into and you must use the seat belt to secure it in place). Depending on your vehicle, you may be able to use the UAS/latch system to secure the car seat to your vehicle. This universal system comes with most new cars and is a special locking device like a seat-belt latch. It works with the latches on all newer baby seats and boosters, so you don't need to use a clamp to hold the seat belt firm. You may also use the seat belt to secure it to your vehicle. Depending on what kind of seat belt you have, you may require a locking clip that often comes with the car seat or booster seat to lock the seat belt. Check in your vehicle manual for instructions.
- Always use the tether strap with a forward-facing car seat that is used with the harness system.
- If you don't understand the manufacturer's instructions, find someone to help you.
- Don't move a child into the next stage of seat too soon. This can lead to injury for a number of reasons. For instance, babies who are moved from a rear-facing car seat to a forward-facing car seat before they

are one year old are at greater risk for serious injury or death in a crash.

- Do not put kids under 12 in the front seat of a vehicle. Evidence overwhelmingly shows that injury to kids is greatly reduced when they sit in the back seat.

And when using your car seat at home, you should be aware of the following:

- Keep car seats on the floor. Babies can and have rocked themselves off counters and tables, so set the car seat on the floor, not on the table.
- Babies can fall over and be suffocated when the car seat is placed on a cushiony surface and tips over, so don't put them on anything soft like a bed or sofa while they are in their car seats.
- Do not use the car seat as a crib. Children have slipped down and suffocated when they got tangled in the straps.

Drowning

We know that the second leading cause of death to Canadian children is drowning. Forty-nine percent of drowning deaths and hospitalizations are a result of swimming pool incidents, open-water occurrences (in lakes or streams) account for about 37 percent, and bathtubs 14 percent. CIHI also tells us that swimming pool deaths and hospitalizations are higher for the youngest age group, newborn to four years, and decrease with age.

One thing is clear from the research: Lack of supervision is a critical factor in drownings. Drowning can occur when a child's hair or body part gets stuck in a drain and the child becomes trapped under the water.

Here are the best ways to ensure your child's water safety:

- Keep a child under 5 within arm's reach when near water. Children over 5 should be closely watched, especially if they cannot swim well. Deaths of 14-year-old children who know how to swim have occurred usually when there is no supervision.
- Install four-sided fencing around swimming pools. It should be at least 4 feet (120 cm) high and have self-closing gates. Safe Kids Canada reports that researchers estimate 7 out of 10 drowning incidents could be prevented with the use of proper fencing for kids under the age of five. Remember that it is not sufficient to close off your backyard. That may protect your neighbours' kids, but you should also consider that access from your house must be controlled as well. Mesh or vertical bars, not horizontal bars, should be used because children can climb horizontal bars.
- When boating, use a properly fitting life jacket. Ninety percent of all recreational boaters who drown in Canada are not wearing life jackets. And remember

to buckle it—some boaters have drowned because they overlooked this simple step. (Remember that even the best swimmer can drown in cold water.)

- Swimming lessons and survival training are very important but they must not be a replacement for supervision.
- Avoid using baby bath seats. These seats—little ring-shaped seats that affix to the bottom of the bath tub—instill a false sense of safety so you feel comfortable leaving the baby in the bath for a few minutes while you leave the room. But the baby can slip down and drown. You may also experience difficulty lifting the baby out of the device if he or she has slipped down. Sometimes the suction cups that hold the seat to the bottom of the tub make it difficult to rip the whole thing up while you're attempting to keep the baby's head up. In other cases, the suction cups don't stick properly at all and the baby slips into the water. In Francesca's experience, bath seats can also lead to injury to the baby's legs. These seats are firm plastic and have no give. Babies' legs tend to stick straight out so getting them into the unit can be painful and lead to injury.
- Despite the fact that Health Canada is reviewing the use of bath seats and has issued a product advisory, we would highly recommend that any parent completely refrain from using that product.

Tip

One of the gifts you can give your children is an ability to swim. It will allow them to enjoy our beautiful country and it may save their lives.

Swimming lessons are as important as driving lessons.

Pedestrian Injury

Pedestrian injury, which can be very severe, is defined as an injury to a pedestrian by a vehicle. Even when children do not die from their injuries, they are often left with long-lasting disabilities. As we saw in the chart, the highest risk of pedestrian injury exists in that five-to-nine age group. This is when kids are mobile and somewhat fearless.

Safe Kids Canada reports that pedestrian injuries occur more in areas where there are

- no formal traffic controls, crosswalks, etc;
- more apartment buildings;
- no formal play areas;
- shared driveways; or
- many cars parked on the curb (impeding drivers' views of kids).

Many of these conditions tend to exist in overcrowded low-income neighbourhoods.

The number-one thing you can do to prevent your children from suffering such injuries is to teach them the rules of the road from a pedestrian viewpoint and to teach them about the many risks associated with playing near moving vehicles of all kinds. While education is important, the best way you can prevent road injury is to combine education with supervision.

Safe Kids Canada's Top Tips Lists

We all know some of the basics of child safety. But often we don't know the precise recommendations for what to look for when we choose products for our kids. The following lists come from a number of brochures and education campaigns of Safe Kids Canada. Contact the organization directly (see the Resource Guide at the end of the chapter) to obtain brochures on these issues and others. They contain much more information and detail—for example, on how to fit your child with a bike helmet.

Top Tips on Avoiding Burns

- Keep kids away from hot food and drinks.
- Make sure that when you have a pot or pan on the stove, the handles don't stick out where kids can grab them.
- Don't remove a pot from a hot stove element. A child could put his or her hand on the element. If the contents of the pot have been removed and it is empty, put some water in it and return it to the hot element until the element cools down.

- Make sure you have a smoke alarm on every level of your house (you need one right outside every bedroom).
- Check smoke alarms once a month.
- Change the batteries in smoke alarms once a year.

Top Tips on Window Safety

- Install a device to stop the window from opening more than 4 inches (10 cm). A child cannot fall through this small a space. A great variety of devices are available to prevent the window opening any wider. Simple measures could include using screws in the window frame to prevent the window from being raised more than 4 inches (10 cm).
- Install a window guard. A window guard forms a barrier in front of an open window. Window guards are sold at hardware and specialty stores and some department stores.
- Keep windows locked if you are not able to use window safety devices.
- Make sure to move furniture away from windows, as well as balcony railings, to prevent young children from climbing up and falling.

Top Tips on Bicycle Safety

- Make sure your child wears a properly fitting helmet. The helmet should not move around on the head and the straps should be snug. You should be able to fit only one finger between the strap and your child's chin. Some of the most serious injuries and deaths are caused by head injury. A helmet reduces the risk of head injury by up to 85 percent.

- Children under 10 should not ride bikes on the road. They just don't have the judgment needed to ride in traffic safely.
- Teach bike safety rules to your child.
- Make sure the bike is the right size and in good working condition: the brakes work well, tires are filled, horns and bells work, etc.

Safe Kids Canada has also published brochures with detailed information on

- safety tips for skateboards, in-line skates, and scooters;
- how to fit your child with a helmet;
- how to know when your child is ready to ride safely;
- biking safely.

Top Tips on Crib Safety

Some babies have died in cribs as a result of getting their heads caught between the bars. Some babies have died in older cribs when the bottom piece that supports the mattress fell down and they got stuck. Other babies have died when their clothing got twisted around one of the posts of the crib—in essence hanging the child until it suffocated. Newer cribs have corrected these design flaws, and that is why the age of a crib is very important.

Here are some key points that you should know regarding cribs:

- Cribs older than 1986 should not be used because they are considered dangerous.
- Crib bars should not be more than 2.5 inches (6 cm) apart.
- Never use a crib without a label that indicates the age of the crib.
- Homemade cribs, while very beautiful, may not be safe to use.

Top Tips on Using Change Tables, High Chairs, and Strollers Safely

- Always ensure that you put the lock on your stroller when the stroller is stopped.
- Make sure that stroller brakes work.
- Use safety straps on strollers and high chairs.
- Never leave your baby alone on the change table. Not only are change tables high, but sometimes they come with straps in which the baby can become entangled.

Top Tips on Keeping Blind and Curtain Cords Safe

- Cut pull cords short and tie them up high.
- Make sure the cords that hold the blind slats in place can't be pulled out more than 6 inches (15 cm). If the cord can be pulled farther than this, throw the blind out—it is not safe.
- Keep your child's furniture far away from blinds.

Top Tips on Baby Walker and Baby Gate Safety

- Baby walkers with wheels: Don't use them. They have been banned for sale in Canada since 2004 because serious injuries have been associated with them.
- Do not use "pressure baby gates" at the top of stairs since a baby can lean on them and fall. At the top of staircases, use baby gates with screws that fasten them to the wall.

Top Tips for Playpen Safety

- Make sure the mesh is the size of a mosquito net. In more open mesh, buttons, hooks, or strings on the baby's clothing can get caught and the baby can die of strangulation.
- Make sure there is nothing close to the playpen that the baby can pull into it (onto its head) or use to climb out.
- Ensure that you have assembled the playpen properly and locked the sides into place so they won't collapse and strangle the baby.

Top Tips on Bunk Bed Safety

There are no laws in Canada to prohibit stores from selling unsafe bunk beds, so you will need to be the regulator on this one!

- Make sure the bunk bed carries a label that shows it meets ASTM standards. ASTM International is an organization that tests consumer and industrial products and creates standards for them. Learn more about them at www.astm.org.

- Guardrails on the top bunk should be no more than 3.5 inches (9 cm) apart.
- Never allow a child younger than six to sleep in the top bunk.

Top Tips on Toy Boxes and Chests

- The lid should be very lightweight or have special hinges that stop it from slamming down on a baby or toddler's head.
- Air holes drilled into the sides and bottom will allow a child who is trapped inside to breathe.

Top Tip on Drawstrings on Children's Clothing

- Drawstrings, especially when located at the head and neck area of clothing, are not safe. Don't buy any clothes with drawstrings. They get caught in things and children can strangle themselves. If you have children's clothing with drawstrings, cut them off.

Top Tips on Playground Safety

Most serious injuries in playgrounds happen as a result of falls from high equipment onto harder surfaces.

- Use playgrounds with a deep, soft surface like sand, wood chips, pea gravel, or rubber.

- No drawstrings on clothing! No helmets with straps either. These can lead to strangulation or tripping.
- If your child is under five, don't let him or her use equipment that is more than 5 feet (1.5 m) from the ground.

Top Tips on Fall Prevention

- Don't use baby walkers with wheels.
- Do not leave babies unattended on high furniture like change tables.
- Use seat belts on items like highchairs and strollers.
- Do not allow your children to play on playground equipment that is too high and meant for older kids (see playground tips).
- Do not use pressure-installed gates on stairways (see baby gate safety).

As your baby becomes a toddler, you'll become aware of the dangers that abound in your seemingly innocent surroundings. Initially, as your baby becomes mobile, he or she will use furniture and fixtures to help pull him- or herself up. Then they discover climbing! The fix is not to toss out your furniture but to be aware of what can happen with different objects in your home. For example, bookcases might need to be securely fastened to a wall, or a delicate sidetable might need to be moved to another location for a few years.

Health Canada has found that injury to children accounts for about $4 billion in health care costs a year.

But the biggest cost cannot be measured in dollars. It is the cost of a life that has been altered forever because of permanent disability. As you review safety concerns in your house, yard, and neighbourhood, you could be saving your child's life. What could be more precious?

RESOURCE GUIDE

ORGANIZATIONS AND ASSOCIATIONS

Safe Kids Canada
www.safekidscanada.ca
Telephone: 1-888-SAFE-TIPS (723-3847)
This organization publishes brochures that are specific to a number of issues affecting child safety, especially safe and unsafe products, home safety, and vehicle safety.

Health Canada—Product Safety
www.hc-sc.gc.ca/cps-spc
Telephone: 1-866-662-0666
Visit this government site to check for product recalls on a regular basis.

B.C. Children's Hospital—Safe Start
www.cw.bc.ca
Telephone: (604) 875-3273
Once you enter the website, click on "Safe Start." You'll find many tips categorized by theme. It will also provide you with the services they offer.

Canadian Institute of Child Health
www.cich.ca
This group provides education, protection, and advocacy to promote children's safety. The most practical part of the website is the links to excellent supports for child care and safety.

Transport Canada
www.tc.gc.ca
Telephone: (613) 990-2309
TTY: 1-888-675-6863
Transport Canada's website has a section on vehicle safety and children. You can find it by clicking on "Child Safety" located directly under the heading "Check It Out."

Canadian Paediatric Society
www.cps.ca
Enter the area for parents and caregivers, which will take you to the Caring for Kids website. This website has a section dedicated to keeping your child safe.

Canadian Red Cross
www.redcross.ca
This site provides information about water and boating safety as well as information on programs offered by the Red Cross such as first-aid courses.

Poison control phone numbers:
Alberta: 1-800-332-1414
British Columbia: 1-800-567-8911
Manitoba: (204) 787-2591
New Brunswick: (506) 857-5555
Newfoundland: (709) 722-1110
Northwest Territories: 1-800-267-1373
Nova Scotia: (902) 428-8161
Prince Edward Island: 1-800-565-8161
Ontario: 1-800-268-9017
Quebec: 1-800-463-5060
Saskatchewan: 1-800-667-4545 or 1-800-363-7474
Yukon: (604) 682-5050
For the hearing impaired: (416) 597-0215

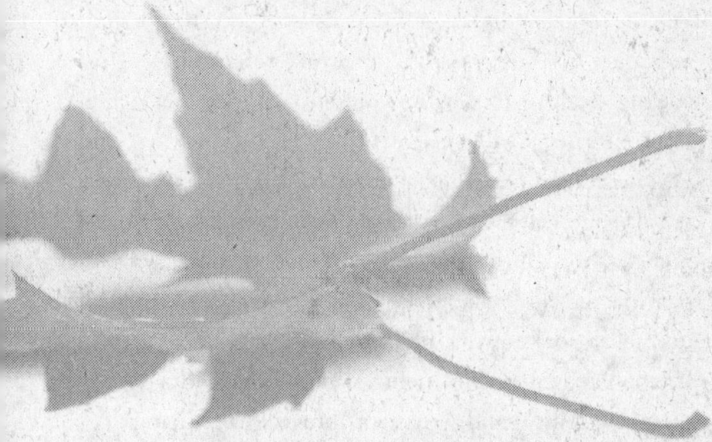

The Middle Years

Statistically speaking, our middle years—from our 20s to our 40s—are our healthiest. Most of our encounters with the health system during those years are for bouts of flu or other occasional illness. Injuries are often from sports or work. However, during the middle years, our eyes, backs, and knees begin to be candidates for repair work!

In these years, our major challenge is to stay healthy and lay the groundwork for a healthy body as we begin to age. What we do in our 20s, 30s, and 40s in the way of exercise, diet, weight, and lifestyle choices interacts with our genetics and shapes our health in later life. As well, we create the habits that determine much of our future health status and even our life expectancy. Chapter 4 is focused on how to get the health system to help us stay healthy. It considers risks to your health and remedies to those risks. The prime responsibility for staying healthy rests with you but you can get some important support.

The remaining two chapters in this section are about navigating health benefits. Both employers and governments, through insurance plans and the tax system, provide an umbrella of coverage. It is not a perfect umbrella, so knowing how it works can benefit you. Chapter 5 focuses on benefits plans and how to navigate their eligibility and payment provisions. Chapter 6 reviews claiming medical expenses on your tax return. The ability of Canadians to recoup health costs not covered by government or employers is not well known. Yet it can be an important source of financial assistance. In our nation there are substantial dollars, over $140 billion per year, available to pay for everything from drugs to doctors to hospitals to mobility aids to home care to eyeglasses and dental. One simple rule is you must claim your benefits to avoid leaving money on the table. Millions of Canadians forgo benefits to which they are entitled out of simple ignorance of their eligibility. Often these plans are complex and need to be understood to be skilfully navigated. Nearly every year the finance minister improves some aspect of the tax system to assist those with medical expenses. Even your accountant, if you have one, may have trouble keeping up. If you are your own accountant, then you really need to keep up!

While we were writing this book, Michael shared some of the ideas with his 21-year-old daughter. He explained the benefits chapter and how many people don't claim their benefits. She said, "Gee, Pops, too bad we don't have a drug plan. I spend a lot of money on prescriptions."

Michael was astonished. "Geneviève, we do have an excellent drug plan. My company plan covers most prescriptions. You are covered."

It turned out that he badly needed to take his own advice. He had never given his daughter the simple plastic card that would save her money on each and every prescription. In fact, the plan covers 80 percent of the cost of most medications. If the co-author of this book is failing to claim benefits, there are likely many others in the same situation.

A happier story occurred when Beryl, one of Michael's co-workers, asked if he knew anything about medical expenses and the tax system. "As a matter of fact I reviewed the chapter just today," he replied. "It's still a draft, but you're welcome to a copy."

The next week Beryl thanked Michael. Her mother's 2005 tax bill had shrunk from $1500 to $300. In addition, her accountant was refiling several previous years of tax returns with hopes of retrieving $3000. In total, Canadians are leaving many millions of dollars on the table in unclaimed benefits. Learn to navigate your benefits plans and the medical-expense-provisions tax system. It will be a profitable journey.

FOUR

Getting the System to Help You Stay Healthy

We are, for the most part, relatively healthy from age 15 to 45. Those 30 years are the years in which we make the least use of health care services. Yet these are the years when we convert our genetic inheritance, through a series of choices we make, into our life expectancy. How we live and the choices we make affect not only how long we will live but in what state of health. The middle years are the years that really shape our outcome. The good thing is that we know a great deal about what has an impact on this conversion process. Our lifestyle, including what we eat and how we exercise, has a huge effect on our health; so too does the environment in which we live. Stress in our workplace or home life can transform into illness.

Most of the history of health care is about treating illness. Most health services are organized to treat sickness. Most money is spent on treatment. Public health has a very different history of preventing illness, but overwhelmingly our attention as a nation has been on access to care. Yet in your middle years, stretching from the teen years to age 50, the key determinants of your health and life expectancy are the choices you make!

Staying Healthy—The Basics

Recently, American health centres have been running full-page ads in Canadian newspapers offering all-body scans, a chance to have your body run through a fancy piece of diagnostic equipment called a positron emission tomography scanner, or a PET. For several hundred or a few thousand dollars, highly qualified personnel will pass you through this machine and then examine all the data that come out. People frequently are curious about whole body scanning, feeling sure this is a great idea. They see it as something like the scanners in *Star Trek*, a chance to find things that the doctor might miss or might not be aware of and potentially save your life. PET scanners do have certain important uses, including locating particularly difficult brain tumours and helping in research that will eventually lead to amazing new discoveries. However, in our view, whole body scanning for people with no sign of illness is an expensive hoax. Occasionally something significant and treatable is found but far more often people are under the illusion that they will live in better health by having the expensive PET scan. The scan may also cause great anxiety about findings that are not indicative of any disease.

In addition, exposing yourself to unnecessary and potentially damaging radiation may do more harm than good. Diagnostic tests should be undertaken only for good scientific and medical reasons. More is not better when it comes to imaging. A single CAT scan to the head is the equivalent of 115 chest X-rays; to the chest, a CAT scan is the equivalent of 400 chest X-rays; and to the abdomen, the equivalent of 500 chest X-rays.

The reality is that for less than 10 dollars another device can provide a much greater support to your longevity. That simple device is a pedometer, a small machine that goes on your belt and measures how many steps you take. A mountain of scientific evidence shows that physical activity is the single most important determinant of your long-term health that you control. Yes, you've inherited the genes, your genetic predisposition from your parents and their parents; yes, there are some genetic diseases that you may be susceptible to—but most of what faces you, such as the possibility of heart disease and diabetes, will be enormously influenced by your level of physical activity. The pedometer allows you to manage how much physical activity you get each day by walking. The recommended dosage is 10,000 steps a day. Other than not smoking, the single best thing you can do is to invest 10 dollars in a pedometer and wear it. You need to determine how active or sedentary the life you lead is. Are you active or are you a couch potato?

Michael has found startling differences based on small changes in behaviour. If he drives from his house to work; goes about his normal daily routine of meetings, presentations, and meals; and drives home, he will be through his day with fewer than 3000 steps. Only one alteration in his routine—to walk the six minutes up the street to take the subway to work and then home—roughly doubles his steps to 6000. Getting off the subway two stops early and walking across the street to his office building—a walk that takes no more than seven minutes—gets him pretty close to his 10,000 allotment for the day. If he needs to make up some steps, an after-dinner walk will accomplish the goal.

So skip the whole body scan—buy a pedometer and get more active. What the middle years are about is organizing your contact with the health system to help you stay healthy—the focus of this chapter. Just as you would invest in routine maintenance to ensure that your automobile lasts beyond the warranty period, so you need to invest to make sure your body will go the distance!

There's no end of interest in keeping you healthy—if you Google "staying healthy in Canada" you get over 3.8 million hits, which include an enormous diversity of advice. The Internet hits run the gamut from the sensible *Canada's Food Guide* to "The Authoritative Guide to Grapefruit Seed Extract"! Nearly everyone wants you to stay healthy: your family, because they care about you; your employer, because they depend on your skills, abilities, hard work, and good health; your government, because it is struggling to find enough dollars to fund our health care system. The health care system, because it has many stresses and strains, would like to treat you later—much later! Only a small number of companies, such as those who make and sell cigarettes and fast food, generally put their profitability ahead of your health. Even in that crowd, salads and healthier foods are being added to the burger-and-fry menus to meet new customer demands.

A March 2006 *Maclean's* magazine poll by the Innovative Research Group noted that 81 percent of Canadians agree that everyone who relies on a public health care system has a responsibility to do their part to stay healthy. So far, the majority of Canadians are still willing to share the financial burden of health care costs even for those who do not take good care of themselves. Only one-third of those surveyed believe that smokers should get a lower priority on waiting lists. Eight in 10 of us still believe the obese should get the same timely access to health care as anyone else. However, 8 in 10 also agree that childhood obesity could overwhelm the health care system in the future. Canadians' future views could shift under those circumstances.

As you approach your middle years, you will find that you are starting to visit health providers more frequently. Your dentist will likely suggest that your routine dental cleaning be done every three or four months instead of six months or annually. Your doctor will have more questions for you at each visit. You may begin to have annual medicals. As well, you will likely find you are getting prescriptions filled more frequently.

There is much you can do to keep yourself in good health. The first and most important aspect of this is to take responsibility for your health. No single step will take you a greater distance toward a healthy life than the one toward greater personal responsibility. Another step is to assemble your care team, which should include your family doctor, with an eye to your longer-term needs. In addition to your team, compiling your health record—not only test results and medication information but insurance coverage and family histories—is essential.

Tip

A few statistics should help convince you of the merits of staying healthy. Based on its National Population Health Survey, Statistics Canada reports that between age 35 and 44, 90 percent of Canadian adults report themselves to be in good or excellent health. By age 65, this drops to 75 percent of Canadian adults. Your goal should be to be able to honestly report yourself to be in good health through the years. After all, misleading Statistics Canada is a serious offence!

There is remarkable consensus on the basic steps involved in maintaining better health. First, there is unanimous scientific opinion that stopping smoking (or not starting) is an effective way of reducing your risk of cancer, heart disease, stroke, and a myriad of other problems. Second, there is agreement that 30 to 60 minutes of moderate exercise each day is good for you. This exercise need not involve weightlifting in a gym. It can be as easy as walking. The third key area is your diet—you are what you eat. To be healthy, you need to eat a balanced diet and a sufficient number of calories. A fourth point is to drink alcohol in moderation. That is it. Those are four basics worth taking seriously.

Tip

Healthful eating advice is easily available compliments of *Canada's Food Guide to Healthy Eating*: www.hc-sc.gc.ca.

Staying healthy will not eliminate the possibility of cancer, heart disease, or stroke, but the above four steps can significantly reduce your risks. You put on a seat belt when you drive not because it eliminates the possibility of accidents but because it increases your chances of survival. You should approach healthy living with the same idea: This will help me live longer and better. The health system can support you with information, coaching, and advice, but the reality is that you are the main determinant of your own health.

Issues surrounding improving your health and looking after our environment are converging. In December 1952, a dense "smoke fog" descended on the city of London, England. By the time it lifted five days later, it had killed more than 4000 Londoners. The city took steps to clean up the high sulphur emissions caused by burning coal that led to the tragedy. And the world gained a new word, the abbreviation of smoke fog to smog.

We seem not to have learned much over the intervening years. In 2005, Toronto had 15 smog alerts covering 53 days. It is estimated that Ontario suffers $10 billion of annual damage linked to polluted air. Of this total, $6.6 billion is attributed to additional health costs, which cover 29 million minor illnesses, 60,000 emergency department visits, 17,000 hospital admissions, and 5800 premature deaths.

Health and environment are indeed the same issue. The population of our planet took thousands of years to reach 1 billion people. Since World War II, it has risen from just over 2.3 billion to 6.5 billion. It is predicted to reach 9 billion by the middle of this century. In 100 years the population will have increased four-fold. This is putting enormous pressure on our environment, but you can take steps to reduce the impact of the deteriorating environment on you. Paying attention to alerts about UV indexes and smog levels is one step. Reducing your own contribution to bad air is another excellent idea.

Let's step back from the large global issues of environment and climate change. What practical steps can you take to arrange the health care and support you will need as you age? What can you do now that will help then?

Tip

Two recent books capture the challenge of climate change driven by air pollution. *An Inconvenient Truth* by former U.S. vice-president Al Gore and *The Weather Makers* by Tim Flannery are more fully described in the Resource Guide at the end of this chapter. Our use of energy has consequences that we need to be aware of. It is clear that we can be part of the solution if we choose to make some changes to how we live.

Your Health Care Team

The foundation on which you should build your health care team is your family doctor. If you live in those parts of Canada where family doctors are not taking new patients—in places such as rural and northern Canada—your alternative may be a nurse-practitioner at a nursing station or community health centre. You'll likely find as you do your research that there is a lot of current emphasis on the "team" aspect of what we now call primary care.

If you cannot find a doctor taking new patients in your area, and you have exhausted your possibilities by contacting the provincial College of Physicians and Surgeons and the medical association, get in touch with your local member of the legislature. Most health care is provincial and our elected members have staff to assist you. Also, look for a community health centre or primary care centre in your area. Staff at these new centres for delivering care may be willing and able to add you to their roster and provide team care. If you are in need of immediate but minor care in a Canadian city, walk-in clinics are advertised in the Yellow Pages. For some Canadians, the walk-in clinic has become their usual place for care. In the north or rural areas, as noted previously, there may be a nursing station or community health centre established by governments to provide care. Asking your local pharmacist for leads on new doctors in town is another good idea.

If you need urgent care, call 911 or go to the emergency department of the nearest hospital. If you need urgent but more minor care, some hospitals have established urgent care clinics either at the hospital or nearby. Getting referred to an urgent care clinic may speed your treatment, as you will not be competing for a busy emergency department doctor's attention with the arriving heart attack and accident victims.

Finding a Family Doctor

Every Canadian should have a family doctor or nurse-practitioner. Most people know about family doctors and what they do, but nurse-practitioners might not be so familiar. Nurse-practitioners can do many things that doctors can do. They can prescribe medications, check for problems, and order many tests. In remote areas like Nunavut, nurse-practitioners are an integral part of the health care system.

Often, books written in other countries contain an entire chapter dedicated to choosing your doctor. Many Canadians have no choice at all. And, where there is a good doctor (family or specialist), they are typically so booked up that a successful appointment is one conducted in sound bites.

A good doctor must be accessible. The reality is that in some parts of this country today you will face a challenge in finding an accessible doctor. In some areas of Canada the supply of family doctors is out of sync with the demand, and doctors are working very long hours just to keep up with their heavy loads.

Tip

Finding a family doctor is not an easy task these days. There is an overall shortage of family doctors in Canada, and in northern and rural areas, shortages can be severe. A number of provincial Colleges of Physicians and Surgeons are trying to help with their on-line "Find a Doctor" service. All the provincial college websites are linked to the Royal College of Physicians and Surgeons of Canada's website, www.rcpsc.medical.org. They are also listed in the Resource Guide at the end of Chapter 14.

Many of us "inherit" our doctors from our parents—we just keep seeing the same doctor our parents took us to when we had colds and needed injections. But in a highly mobile country such as ours, the search for a new family doctor is—or should be—part of getting settled in a new community. The best way to find a doctor is through word of mouth. If you know someone who is happy with their doctor, you can ask if the doctor is taking on new patients, then call the doctor's office and book an appointment. If he or she is not taking new patients and your friend or neighbour has been a long-time patient, they can ask the doctor on your behalf if he or she would make an exception and take you on. This is typically a more successful tactic if your friend is not a difficult patient. If you have a choice between a doctor who has an opening in his or her practice and one who doesn't but would agree to take you on, and you hear that both are good, go for the doctor who has an opening. You stand more of a chance of having access when you need it.

If you are lucky enough to live in an area with enough doctors to offer a choice, take into account the type of facilities the doctors have. Some doctors have ultrasound facilities or X-ray facilities nearby. More important, it is great to have a pharmacy and a lab located very close to your doctor (maybe even in the same building). Family doctors are now beginning to practise more and more in groups that work as teams. This means that you may have access to a doctor when yours is not available or after office hours. This is definitely something you should ask about. Newer practices are incorporating nurses and other practitioners. The nurses take on functions that they are qualified to do, freeing up the doctors' time to do what they are trained to do.

Once you've chosen your doctor, arrange to have your medical records transferred to his or her office. Don't wait for the doctor to do this. When you need to visit your doctor, your records will be handy for review.

It's important to make good use of the time you spend with your family doctor. In order to maximize your visit, no matter the reason, take the following with you:

- A list of your questions
- A pen and paper to take notes

Tip

Tell the doctor why you are taking notes! You will discover that note-taking is a major theme of this book, yet we had never considered the doctor's interpretation of the patient taking notes. Since we have interviewed several physicians, we now know it is good practice to explain to the doctor up front why you are doing this. The doctor may think that you are creating a record in case he or she messes up. Explain clearly that you may need to go somewhere else and it may be helpful to have a record of what this visit yields.

Compile your list of questions between appointments as issues come up. Don't wait till the night before to try to remember your questions—chances are, you won't be able to summon them. Leaving out a detail of a symptom might have significant implications on your care.

Once you've chosen your doctor, you may need to manage your expectations about the amount of time he or she will give a patient who is low risk and doing fine. Visits to the doctor are not like a social tea party. Most books talk about finding a doctor you can "talk to." Don't forget that this is in relation to what you are seeing the doctor about, not cocktail party chit-chat. If you have a question, an issue, a problem, or a concern directly related to your condition, you do need to be able to relate well to your doctor. But if "talk" means sharing your knowledge about the developmental phases of a fetus or last night's hockey game, a doctor with a waiting room full of patients may get a little edgy. Some physicians have nurse-practitioners who will provide support and answers to many of your questions. And, as we will see, there are other health care professionals who can also assist you in their areas of expertise.

Finally, remember that just because a doctor may seem a little cut and dried and to the point, that doesn't mean that he or she is not competent. It just means that you will need to work harder as a patient to ensure that your concerns and questions are answered.

Getting the Tests You Need

Your family doctor is your key resource in getting the tests you need. Your first important step is to ensure that your doctor knows your medical history and the medical history of your family. The timing of a number of tests is dependent on family history. If you have no family history of colon cancer, for example, getting a colonoscopy in your 50s is recommended. If one or more family members had colon cancer, it may be a hereditary condition with a genetic cause. If your doctor is aware of this, you will likely be tested earlier and more frequently. If you have symptoms, tests are ordered to determine a diagnosis. A reluctance to admit a symptom can harm your care and outcome by delaying testing. A full and honest disclosure to your doctor is vital.

Pragmatist or Purist?

Francesca likes to tell of a conversation she had with Dr. Reg Kusnierczyk, a pillar of the Sudbury medical community. He claims there are two types of doctors: the Purist and the Pragmatist. The Purist will not prescribe anything until all the tests have been done, the results are in, the bug isolated, and the X-ray read. The Purist does it by the book.

If you live in a big urban centre where labs, doctors, hospitals, after-hour clinics, and diagnostic equipment are readily available, the Purist is a great doctor to have. Those who live in smaller, underserviced communities may prefer the category Dr. Kusnierczyk calls "the Pragmatist." This doctor understands that in a place of limited resources, the Purist methodology may not always be practical.

Francesca's mother, who suffers from multiple sclerosis, provides a good example of how this type of doctor works. She can run into trouble when a minor cold settles and festers. It can turn from a virus into a bacterial infection fairly quickly, and she will be unable to get out of bed. Because her limbs become stiff and won't support her body weight, she cannot walk, making it impossible to take her to the doctor.

People like Francesca's mother need the Pragmatist type of doctor. It is this doctor who will say to her, "I don't hear a chest infection but this is a long weekend and given your history and complications, I'll write you a prescription. Don't have it filled unless you're running a fever or are wheezing." The Purist would die a thousand deaths at this practice. But in underserviced areas, it is often the way the Pragmatist doctor needs to practise medicine. If you live in a remote or underserviced area where getting to see someone who can write a prescription is difficult, or if you have a complex medical history or a medical condition that makes it impossible for you to move when you get really sick, you will fare better with the Pragmatist than you will with the Purist.

Beyond Your Doctor

Some of your care team will flow directly from your family doctor or family health team, based on your needs at the time. Other members of your health team, such as your pharmacist, may come from your local neighbourhood. Over a period of years, others may be added, such as a physiotherapist or a nutritionist.

It is important that you see your team for the value it will bring to your longer-term health. Too often we interact with the health system only when we are ill and need care, but establishing relationships with people such as your pharmacist now will be an advantage if you become ill.

It may sound odd, but your employer can be part of your team. Many employers offer active programs to improve employees' health. Your employer wants you healthy, if not wealthy. Check out what is available in the way of health promotion at your workplace and what you are eligible to benefit from. Employers can be allies in maintaining your health and enhancing your well-being.

Assembling Your Own Health Record

We live in the age of technology. Automated teller machines spit out cold hard cash based on a plastic card. Our identities can be stolen from the Internet. You get on a plane based on a boarding pass issued from a machine in the airport. Trillions of dollars in investments exist as data in cyberspace. It might surprise you to know, then, that much information is still in paper record form. For example, your health information is a paper record, most often stored in a variety of locations. Part of your health record is likely in a paper file at the office of your family doctor. The local pharmacy may have an electronic record of your prescriptions. One hospital may have X-rays and printed test results from that bout of pneumonia you suffered. Another hospital may have the paper record of your colonoscopy. It is extremely likely that the full picture of

Tip

Many pharmacies, such as Shoppers Drug Mart through its HealthWatch program, provide a great deal of information on prescription drugs. Shoppers HealthWatch program provides an automatic warning of drug-to-drug interactions and provides patients with a great deal of information on the medication prescribed.

your health history, including records of tests and treatments, is not available in one place.

Until this scattered method is improved, the onus is on you to assemble and manage your own records. It's not as hard as it might sound, but it can take some perseverance on your part. Gather all records for your family doctor. Ask for duplicates of test results and even insurance medicals so your family doctor can have a complete record. Keep a copy of all records for yourself and your family, as well. Remember the evacuees from New Orleans who lost all records in the flood. Better to have them in two places, your home and your doctor's office.

Your health file should contain the following:

- Diagnostic tests such as blood tests, blood pressure readings, EKGs (electrocardiograms) and any X-rays, CT scans, MRIs (magnetic resonance imaging), or PETs (positron emission tomography)
- A list of all prescription medications, along with notes on minor and major adverse reactions
- Family medical history

Tip

Be sure you include in your record all the medications you're taking. There can be dangerous side effects or interactions among various drugs, whether they are natural or chemically manufactured.

- Insurance medicals conducted for personal or employer insurance
- Immunization records
- Hospitalization records and details of any surgery
- Dental records
- Health insurance documents

A handy aid to help you keep track of all this is some software called the Body Journal, which allows you to store and update the health records for your whole family on your home or office computer. It allows you to record all doctors' appointments, to monitor health conditions, and to provide access through an emergency health card to any doctor treating you. The Body Journal comes with a handy health handbook. Further information is provided in the Resources section at the end of this chapter.

On a larger scale, to bring some order and rationalization to the rather scattered approach we described earlier, a corporation called Canada Health Infoway has entered into a partnership with the provinces and the health delivery system to solve the problem. Its goal is to get 50 percent of Canadians an electronic health record by 2010. However, without further investment by governments and health organizations, it may well be 2020 before we all have an accessible electronic health record. During those 14 long years, you are well advised to assemble your own record as described above and keep it handy for doctor and hospital visits.

Tip

To find out more about Canada Health Infoway and its mandate, go to www.infoway-inforoute.ca.

An illustration of the benefits of electronic records is related on the Infoway website. It illustrates how the Pharmaceutical Information Network (PIN) is working in Alberta. This system links community doctors, pharmacists, hospitals, and other health care providers and gives them access to a patient's confidential medication history. The example given is of Matilda, a 75-year-old woman who was having problems with her memory and was taken to the doctor for assessment. When the doctor asked her what medications she was taking, Matilda couldn't name any drugs she was taking or who might have prescribed any. The doctor was able to access her electronic health record, where he discovered that some of her medications could be responsible for her memory loss. He was also able to get the results of lab tests performed on Matilda over the previous year, helping him to assemble a fully formed picture of her health status and to continue treatment without any duplication or risk.

If you live in Alberta, you can follow the example of Matilda and go a step farther—you can access your own health records, a right that was granted by the Health Information Act in 1999. But if you are in a province that is not as far along the road to electronic pharmaceutical records, you need to do it yourself.

Finally, a lot of attention has been placed on the question of privacy of health information in Canada. Privacy is an important issue but so too is access to your health information to assist your treatment. Keeping your own record is one sound way of keeping health professionals fully informed and maintaining control over your privacy. First, it is important to realize that paper health records are not perfectly secure. Paper records can be lost, stolen, or accidentally thrown in the garbage. Every few years the Canadian media carries a story about paper records being misplaced. Sometimes a doctor dies and records are wrongly tossed in the local Dumpster. After the paper records blow down Main Street, a furor ensues.

Electronic heath records are protected by privacy legislation at both the federal and provincial levels. The key methods of ensuring privacy are to remove personal identifiers from data in large health databases and to receive consent from patients to the gathering and use of their personal health information. This permission can be refused by patients.

Records can start quite simply, with that pencil and paper we recommended earlier that you take to your doctor's appointment so you can write down what the doctor tells you. Keeping careful track of the advice you have been given is very important if you have a long-standing health problem or condition, especially if your condition is unusual and capable of being misdiagnosed. Beth Grosso, Francesca's sister, provided an excellent story of her own to illustrate this point and the general point about the importance of keeping records.

> I have had to deal with major vision problems all my life. I have seen many specialists and have learned a little about navigating the system from my experiences and mistakes.
>
> Quite often, I would be sitting in the office of an eye specialist and would get asked the question, "So, tell me about your eyes." What a question! Where would I even begin? It soon became obvious that no doctor had a complete file on me.
>
> I never considered this to be a big deal. I felt that as long as I was there to fill people in, everything was fine. I was wrong. At one point, my ophthalmologist's practice became very specialized and I no longer fit the criteria to be his patient. I already had an optometrist, but he told me that someone like me needed an ophthalmologist as well. Finding one was not an easy task. In order to see an ophthalmologist, I needed someone to write a convincing referral letter. Because I had seen so many different eye doctors, no one doctor could do this. Not even my optometrist had my complete history.

I finally did manage to see an ophthalmologist. This is because quite a few years prior to all this, my dad, worried that I had a detached retina, took me to see one of his colleagues on Christmas Eve. Although that doctor didn't discover a detached retina, my dad asked him for a letter describing what he did see. He asked him to include some of my eye history in this letter so we could have it down on paper. Years later, it was that letter that provided the history I needed to get me in to see an ophthalmologist.

I learned a few things from this. I now ask doctors for copies of letters that they are sending other doctors with regard to my eyes. I have learned that if I don't ask, I won't get them. Also, if I ever forget to ask the specialist, I can always ask my family doctor. I didn't realize that she has every single piece of correspondence about my eyes in my file in her office. She gets copies of nearly everything. When I found this out, I asked her if I could have copies of any letter related to my eyes. I also gave her a copy of the letter from the doctor who saw me Christmas Eve (she didn't have that one). I have also got in touch with the eye doctor who took care of me when I was a kid. He came by one day with not only letters, but all his clinical notes as well.

Asking for copies of letters not only helps you start building a "file" but also helps clarify exactly what is going on as you are being treated. I was recently sent to an eye specialist who wanted to order an "a-scan" on my eyes. I had no clue what an "a-scan" was and I probably would have forgotten the test name soon after my appointment. However, because I asked my doctor to give me a copy of the letter he was going to write, I was well aware of the test he ordered—and it was a good thing, too. When I showed up to have my "a-scan" done, I was asked if I was ready for my cataract surgery. I laughed, thinking these people had a real sense of humour. I soon realized that they had no clue why I was there. I had to tell them. I learned something else from this. Sometimes, it is not good enough to ask for a copy of a letter. Now, I actually write stuff down while I am in the doctor's office or as soon as I get home.

I have also learned to go into a doctor's office with notes. I learned this from my experiences with my eyes as well. For years, I was noticing how night blind I was and how my visual field seemed to be getting smaller. I mentioned this a few times to some eye doctors but obviously did not mention it as often as I should have. A couple of years ago, I was seen by a retina specialist. He had never seen me before in his life, and I was trying to give him the *Reader's Digest* abridged version of my eye troubles. I totally forgot about mentioning those two main symptoms. After he looked in my eyes, he asked me about night blindness and visual field loss. That is when I told him just how much I suffered from this. He then started the testing needed to see if I had retinitis pigmentosa [RP, a hereditary retinal disease that leads to progressive loss of visual field and night vision]. Off I went to get an ERG [an electroretinogram, which is a test that is used to diagnose the disease] done. As it turns out, I seem to have some form of RP. The people at the clinic were surprised that I was an adult but had never had an

ERG. I wondered if, had I taken a written list of symptoms to earlier doctors' appointments, I would have got the ERG sooner.

A final thing I have learned is that the person who knows my eyes the best is me. I am learning that sometimes I need to stand up for myself in a doctor's office. Once when I arrived at the office of a retina specialist for an appointment, I forgot my lens case and because of this was told that I could not be seen. As I left the office, I tried to rebook for the next week, but I was told I had to wait a year because OHIP had already been billed. I felt there was nothing I could do, so I rebooked for the next year. When I told this to my sister, she told me to call the doctor's office and remind them why I was being seen in the first place. I didn't think it would help, but I left a message anyway. My sister was right. The specialist must have been under the impression that I was just there for a checkup, which is why there was no urgency to rebook. The secretary was probably going by standard procedure of waiting a year from the last time OHIP was billed. Once I reminded them, they made an appointment immediately.

Tip

One advantage of having your own health record is that it will give you the confidence to ask the questions that you or your advocate needs to ask.

RESOURCE GUIDE

BOOKS

An Inconvenient Truth. Al Gore (New York: Rodale, 2006).

Former Vice-President Al Gore's film has a companion book of the same title and it is a must-read. In particular his section entitled "So Here's What You Personally Can Do to Help Solve the Climate Crisis" (pages 304–321) is a worthwhile have-to-do-something guide.

The Weather Makers. Tim Flannery (New York: HarperCollins, 2005).

Equally powerful is Tim Flannery's book. Chapter 35, "Over to You," is a guide to steps you can take to improve the environment.

SOFTWARE

Body Journal
bodyjournal.com.
This software has been developed to allow you to store information about your health and health care on computer or PDA. Everything from test results to statistics on weight can be stored for each family member. The information can also be shared with your doctor or other care providers. The program also links you to on-line health information.

GOVERNMENT PROGRAMS

HealthyOntario.com
Ministry of Health, Ontario
www.healthyontario.com

BC HealthGuide
Ministry of Health, British of Columbia
www.bchealthguide.org

You don't have to be a resident of Ontario or British Columbia to benefit from these terrific resources. The Ontario website provides a wide array of information and tips on staying healthy.

Health Canada
Canada Food Guide to Healthy Eating and Physical Activity
www.hc-sc.gc.ca

Public Health Agency of Canada
www.phac-aspc.gc.ca
This relatively new agency provides a series of Canadian Physical Activity Guides tailored to youths, adults, and seniors. Their website has more information.

Regional Health Organizations
In all provinces but Ontario and Prince Edward Island, regional health authorities manage health services. Ontario has recently established Local Health Integration

Networks (LHINs), but they are in their early stages. The implication of this reform is that much authority has moved from provincial governments and from individual hospitals and health services to the region. The regional organization has responsibility both for the health of the population in its area and for caring for those who become ill. The aim is to provide much greater integration of health services so that patients can be guided from one part of the system to another rather than being lost on the way. Progress has been achieved, but there is still a need for patients to be informed and to take responsibility for navigating. Your LHIN's website is a good place to acquaint yourself with the services available.

An excellent example of this new world of Canadian health care delivery is the Capital Health region in Edmonton:

Capital Health
Edmonton, Alberta
www.capitalhealth.ca/EspeciallyFor/weightwise
Telephone: (780) 408-LINK (5465) or 1-866-780-5465
Capital Health, an integrated health system, has a weight-management program called WeightWise—Healthy Weight for Healthy Lives. Visit their website for information about their workshops and other advice.

FIVE

Navigating Your Benefits Plans

When people talk about health care in Canada, much of the discussion centres on the role of government. It is true that governments pay 70 percent of the total bill for health care, with the other 30 percent paid by private insurance or out of pocket by Canadians; that is, of the $142 billion spent in Canada annually, almost $100 billion comes from government tax revenues—contributed by you, the taxpayer. Governments pay 99 percent of doctors' bills in Canada and over 90 percent of hospital bills, but when it comes to dentists, drugs, eyeglasses, hearing aids, nursing care, physiotherapy, and other health services, individual Canadians get only partial support from government. For these services, we rely heavily on special government programs, employer-sponsored health care plans, and plans that we privately purchase on our own.

As with any insurance, government and private plans contain a host of details and requirements that can make the difference between getting all, more, less, or no reimbursement. How much you get depends on what the plans cover. This is particularly true for government-sponsored plans. It also depends on how you file your claim, which is especially true for private plans.

This chapter will provide you with an overview of what is available in the way of health insurance plans and how they work, along with some tips on how to get the most out of them. Navigating increasingly complex benefit plans is a skill you're going to need. We'll help you learn how to acquire it in this chapter.

In Canada there are three basic categories of health insurance:

- Medicare insurance is the public health insurance plan that covers services like hospital stays and physician services, and tests and procedures deemed medically necessary. The cost is covered by government. Medicare is accessible when you have a valid provincial or territorial health card and is available to all Canadians and residents of Canada. Most important, hospital services and the physicians' services and drugs you use while you are in hospital are covered. Other services are provided beyond these, but they vary by jurisdiction. If you move from one province or territory to another and you have been receiving medical care, be sure to check which of your treatments and medicines are covered. You do not have to fill out paperwork or file claims for reimbursement. Showing your provincial or territorial health insurance card is sufficient to receive most services.

- Public plans and special government-sponsored insurance plans that cover populations with special needs are the second category. These will be referred to in this chapter as "public plans," but they are not to be confused with general medicare-insured services described above because they are not available to all Canadians or residents. A good example would be drug insurance for seniors, which covers items most people would pay for out of pocket unless they have a private insurance plan.
- Private plans, the third category, include employer-sponsored plans (health insurance provided by corporations and governments to their employees) and plans purchased by individuals.

This chapter will cover two of these categories of insurance. We will not spend much time discussing medicare since it is well covered in other chapters, although we will touch on medicare eligibility for new residents and loss of medicare coverage when you are out of the country for extended periods of time.

The categories of insurance we are focusing on are important supplements to health care coverage in Canada. While we may believe that all our health needs are covered under medicare, or hope that someday they

Tip

For Canadian patients in hospitals, all drug costs are covered. When a patient leaves a hospital, sometimes it's possible to arrange for two or four weeks' supply of the medication. In some cases, with oral antibiotics and certain other drugs, that will be all that is needed for the patient to be restored to health. It is certainly worth having a conversation with the doctor who is attending you in the hospital about drugs you will be taking after the hospital stay.

all will be, this is not now the case. As a result, Canadians often rely on a combination of plans, such as those provided by employers or private health care insurers, to cover their needs.

Many people judge the value of their benefits plan by how well it covers prescription medications. Medications are a big-ticket item, and they are used more and more frequently by more and more people as scientists discover ways of controlling or stopping diseases through medication rather than in an operating room. As a nation we spend more on drugs than we do on doctors—each year since 1997, the total bill for drugs has climbed faster than the total bill for doctors. In health care, drugs are now the number-two spending item for Canadians, second only to hospital costs. Prescription drugs cost the Canadian health system about $18 billion per year. It is staggering to think that drug expenses are growing at a rate of 10 percent per year. It's clear then why most people put a priority on how well the cost of medications are covered when they are assessing an insurance plan.

Navigating for the Uninsured

Nine percent of Canadians are considered underinsured and another 2 percent have no drug insurance at all. Many of these Canadians have children who therefore aren't covered enough to meet their health care needs. If you are in this category, here are a few tips:

- If you are paying for drugs out of your own pocket, the hospital pharmacy may be a lower-cost alternative than a retail pharmacy.
- Ask your doctor whether you can get a prescription for a longer period of time, such as 90 days, to reduce the cost to you. Each time you go back to the pharmacy, you pay a dispensing fee. If your prescription is for a longer period of time, you cut down on the trips and dispensing fees.
- Cut out dispensing fees. Some pharmacies—Wal-Mart is one—do not charge a dispensing fee, which is a fee generally charged by pharmacists for their skill and labour. The rest of the prescription price is made up of the cost of the drug and the pharmacy's mark-up.
- If you can, buy some private insurance. Private insurers offer many packages so you can purchase what you need, but be sure to do your homework.
- Tell your doctor you have no insurance. Doctors usually give patients free samples or will prescribe a less expensive generic. See the tip on generics.

Public Plans

Who They Cover

As we said earlier, public plans are government-sponsored plans that don't fall within the mandate of medicare. These public plans, which are most often drug plans, are mainly directed at those individuals who either have less ability to pay for prescription drugs and likely do not have a private plan or are in need of key treatments and are afflicted with conditions for which drug costs are prohibitively high. Public plans infrequently cover other health services for very vulnerable populations like seniors; however, these programs tend to be very limited in scope. It is wise to check with your province or territory to see what you may be eligible for besides medications and to find out whether you fit in one of the above-listed categories. Public coverage varies widely across the country, with some provinces having much more comprehensive coverage than others.

Public plans typically provide coverage for

- Vulnerable populations such as welfare recipients and seniors;
- Adults and children for important immunizations (all provinces have immunization programs that cover children, and most cover adults for things like flu vaccines);
- People who have certain catastrophic diseases that require very costly drug therapy (Ontario, for instance, has the Trillium Drug Program), although

not all jurisdictions have good catastrophic drug programs;
- First Nation and Inuit Canadians (covered by the federal government).

Public drug plans will reimburse all or a part of the costs associated with drugs for individuals who are eligible under these programs. While all provinces and territories offer drug programs, there is little consistency in what is offered, now, and to whom. Government drug programs for children are far less comprehensive than programs for seniors. If you have been diagnosed with any condition whose treatment will cost you money, it will be well worth the effort to find out if there is financial help for you. Organizations have been created to disseminate information and aid to sufferers of conditions such as cancer, multiple sclerosis, and diabetes (and many others). Your doctor or nurse can give you information about such organizations. Contacting them is an important first step, not only in understanding your condition but also in finding out what supports are available to you for little or no cost.

What's Covered?

All provincial and territorial plans cover only those medications that are on the list, or formulary, that has been approved by the province. Though there are a number of reasons that a drug may not be included on the formulary, cost considerations tend to heavily influence formulary decisions. Some provinces have a mechanism by which a prescriber such as a doctor can apply to have a medication covered for his or her patient even if it isn't on the formulary; however, these mechanisms tend to be somewhat cumbersome. Frequently these situations are dealt with on a case-by-case basis but some jurisdictions have special clauses that allow for extraordinary cases. These exceptions are typically not advertised. Your doctor would need to request special consideration, and hopefully he or she would know how to get the ball rolling. However, in the event that he or she doesn't, get in touch with your ministry of health's drug programs branch, and ask if there is any mechanism to get special consideration.

Pharmaceutical companies fight hard to ensure that their products are listed on the government formularies. Frequently, brand-name pharmaceutical products are replaced on government formularies by less expensive generic products once the patent protection on the brand-name medication is over. This is called "generic substitution" (see Tip, page 147). In many provinces, seniors' drug plans promote substituting brand-name medications with generic medications when possible. They do this by covering only up to a certain amount, usually the cost of the least expensive product. However, if individuals wish to have the brand-name medication, they can pay the difference.

In some provinces, there is mandatory substitution, meaning that if there is a less expensive medication

Tip

A further way of navigating the high cost of prescription drugs is to understand a bit about the world of generic drugs. Generic drugs, sometimes called knock-offs, are drugs made by companies and produced for sale after the patent period expires on the original drug. They are often priced substantially below the cost of the original drug and are regulated to be the same chemical entity—that is, the same active ingredients are in the generic pill as were in the original brand-name pill. Ask your pharmacist when presenting the prescription whether there is a generic equivalent. Your pharmacist is likely to have on hand a good supply of the generic drug. They almost certainly will save you money.

deemed by the government to be an acceptable substitution, it must be dispensed instead of the more expensive medication.

Generic substitution has caused a number of legal and public relations wars between governments and drug manufacturers, who argue that while medications may be the same or similar in therapeutic content (active ingredients), there may be differences in the way they are administered and absorbed into the body. One of the more persuasive arguments made against generic substitution is that there may be differences in dosage and dosage times, which could cause confusion for the patient who has been on a different medication schedule. It may lead to the patient's not taking the medication properly. Here, it is argued, seniors tend to be the most at risk.

Tip

Be very certain of the dosage you need to take and when. Invest in some of those handy pill boxes that let you organize your medication by time of day, day of the week, or other configurations. In addition, make your pharmacist your best friend—he or she can guide you through confusing changes.

Public Drug Programs for Seniors

In Chapter 10, "Navigating Health Care for Seniors," we provide an overview of public drug programs for people over 65. You should know that no matter which province or territory you live in, it has a drug plan for you once you turn 65. The details and financial arrangements of these plans differ from jurisdiction to jurisdiction. For the most part, seniors participate in these programs because it is worth their while to do so. Many provinces charge no premium and have reasonable deductibles. However, in some jurisdictions, access barriers such as premiums make it too costly for seniors to participate. Furthermore, in some provinces, seniors are subject to income tests. Many seniors are considered ineligible to participate in government drug insurance plans because they don't satisfy the low income requirement.

Public Drug Plans for Children

Overall, government plans spend relatively little (only 1.2 percent of their drug expenditures) on programs for children under 14, despite needs for medications. This low figure doesn't mean that children require fewer prescription medications. When children are very young, they need a whole host of vaccinations, and indeed many are covered. However, not all vaccines that are recommended by the Canadian Paediatric Society are covered in each province and territory.

Children also frequently go from having a bad viral infection to acquiring a bad bacterial infection that requires antibiotics. And just as there are diseases that affect seniors more than the general population, so too are there diseases that affect children more than adults. Some are very serious. Others are not serious when addressed in a timely manner, but they can be very costly.

An article by Wendy Ungar, a senior scientist at the Hospital for Sick Children in Toronto, and Maciej Witkos points out that while provinces agree on the importance of providing medication benefits to seniors (governments spend about 65 percent of their drug expenditures on seniors), "there is no agreement on the importance to provide the same benefits to other vulnerable populations, including Canada's 7.5 million children." They comment that the low provincial drug spending for children may reflect a lack of government-sponsored programs to meet children's needs and is not proof that children have fewer drug needs. While immunizations are generally covered (see Chapter 2), drugs for children often are not. Also, many childhood diseases require parents to pay out of pocket or

Tip

The discrepancy between how the provinces administer drug plans for children and adults is huge. Check which programs are available and which drugs are covered in your province or territory by visiting your provincial ministry of health website. If your child has a serious condition, it may be worth moving, even though it seems a drastic solution. An Ontario mother whose child could not receive government supports for autism because of his age decided to move to Alberta, where these programs are covered.

take out private insurance if they have no other coverage. There is a real patchwork across the country and you will need to talk to your doctor about available medication public programs if your child is faced with a serious illness or condition. Alternatively, you can contact your provincial ministry of health, drug programs branch.

Sadly, your access to a prescription drug under a provincial program is often determined by where you live, rather than by how badly your child needs the drug. All provinces and one territory, Nunavut, have drug programs that provide benefits to children for those on social assistance. You can ask the nurse in the nursing station how to apply or contact the territorial government. But if your child suffers from a serious chronic disease, there is little consistency in public drug plans.

The conclusion by Ungar and Witkos is succinct and valid: "All children across Canada, no matter what province they call home, are entitled to ready and affordable access to the same, comprehensive formulary of medications." Policy-makers, please take note!

Public Drug Plans for Low-Income Earners

All provinces agree that people on social assistance must have provincial drug coverage. They don't agree on what kind of coverage should be offered for low-income families who don't qualify for social assistance. The result is that in many provinces, the working poor are left with little or no coverage. Their employers are too small or poor to provide an employer drug plan. And, when it comes to cost-sharing with the patient, low-income earners will find there are big discrepancies in which provincial drug plans and programs they qualify for. There are even differences within a province, depending on the drug program for which you qualify. Some provinces have deductibles or premiums or co-payments;

Tips

If you cannot afford the drug, deductible, or co-payment, speak to the person prescribing your medication. You may be prescribed an alternative product that is lower in price but just as effective.

If a doctor offers you a free sample and you can afford your medication, turn it down, telling your doctor you prefer it to be available to someone who really needs it. If we all do our part, we can help improve access to costly drugs for someone less fortunate.

others have combinations of these; and only one province, Newfoundland, has no cost-sharing.

These out-of-pocket expenses can be significant, making it very difficult for part-time workers or low-income families to access prescription medicines. The bottom line is that provincial drug plans and real estate have one thing in common: location, location, location.

Tip

Know your eligibility for government programs by contacting your province or territory's ministry of health. Do not assume that your jurisdiction covers the same things as another. You'll find the programs they offer on their website. See the Resource Guide at the end of the book for web addresses.

Private Insurance Plans

The Canadian Institute for Health Information reported in *Explaining the 70/30 Split: How Canada's Health Care System Is Financed* that in 2002 Canadian health insurance plans paid out $14 billion for claims and administration of claims. Of this total, two-thirds was for drug and dental care. Clearly these are two key areas covered by private plans. These plans cover things that are not covered by medicare.

Private insurance can be offered by your employer or purchased by you on your own. The federal government provides a benefits plan to those in the military and to its employees as well. Provincial and territorial governments also provide their employees with plans. These aren't "public plans"—they are the same as employer plans.

Canadians who have purchased their own private health insurance have often done so either because they do not have an employer-sponsored plan or because they want to supplement their employer-sponsored plan with better coverage. For example, if you work for a company that offers health care but not dental care, you can purchase your own dental benefits.

Different types of health insurance are emerging, such as critical-care illness insurance and long-term care insurance. Here is a list of some of the products offered to individuals wanting to purchase their own private health insurance:

- General health, drug, and dental insurance
- Practitioners such as chiropractors, massage therapists, opticians, dietitians (as a group generally referred to as allied health professionals)
- Medical devices
- Critical illness insurance
- Long-term care insurance
- Out-of-country health insurance

To purchase private health insurance, generally you need to be a resident of Canada and covered by medicare. Insurance companies will want to assess you to find out your health status and your needs. Based on this information, they may limit the amount and type of insurance you can get. They can also put restrictions on the types of medications or services that they will provide. For example, if you are currently taking a regular prescription medication, they may exclude that medication from your coverage. You will need to check what you are eligible for. Also, your premiums may increase or you may not be insured at all if you have certain medical conditions or are over a certain age.

Employer-sponsored plans and plans you purchase on your own operate in much the same way. Many employer plans typically offer a standard package of benefits spanning a number of items. Some employer plans offer more custom packages where the employee can choose different benefits. Plans you purchase on your own can be full-coverage packages or targeted-benefit plans that are, for example, geared to just medications or just dental. In employer benefit plans, the employer usually pays a percentage of the premium and you pay the rest. Some employers cover 100 percent of the premium, though this is no longer the norm. Others cover 80 percent, and many cover 60 percent of the premium.

Tip

Remember that the premium the employer pays is a taxable benefit to you. The premium you pay can be claimed as a medical tax credit on your income taxes (see Chapter 6).

Employer Benefit Plans

Most employer plans cover certain basic benefits apart from prescription drugs and dental. It is very important to be aware of what these other benefits are. Often people are keenly aware of the coverage they will receive on prescription medications or dental. But they don't really bother with the other miscellaneous items that can be important. Among these is coverage for a private or semi-private room for a hospital stay. Under this coverage, if you require surgery or are giving birth to a child, your hospital will have an option of placing you in a room by yourself or with one other person rather than in a ward room with many other patients. If you know you will be entering hospital for treatment, be sure to make arrangements with the hospital for a private or semi-private room as soon as possible. These accommodations tend to be filled quickly in older facilities.

If you are nearing retirement or are planning to leave an employer, you need to know what carry-forward provisions exist, if any. In some cases, retiree benefits are very generous; in other cases, once you've left active work your benefit plan changes.

You should also be aware of yearly ceilings on your benefits. For instance, in the case of dental, you may be allowed only a certain number of procedures per year. See page 171 for more detail about dental coverage.

Speak to a representative of the insurance company or your human resources department if you have questions.

Be informed! Understanding your plan can greatly influence the cost and benefits you derive from it.

Tip

If you work for a large employer, there are likely to be seminars offered by that employer—sometimes even during working hours—where you can get a better understanding of your benefit plan from personnel who work in the human resources department. There may even be an employee benefits information package on the website that you can print out to keep for reference.

Keep all your "Explanation of Benefits" statements from your employer. Any portion of a claim that is not paid by your insurer can be claimed on your income tax (see Chapter 6, "Claiming Medical Expenses").

Medical Savings Accounts

In recent years, some insurance companies have switched from conventional benefit plans to something called medical savings accounts, or medical spending accounts. They shift the burden of decision-making onto you, the employee, or the plan beneficiary. They generally come with a maximum dollar figure for the amount you can spend. You can spend that money on drugs, dental, or eyeglasses. When you reach the end of the allotted amount, you have no further ability to claim until the next year. The idea is to turn plan beneficiaries into smart shoppers. There is some evidence that the medical savings account can work to the advantage of both employers and individual plan participants because it means that for a defined amount paid by the employer, the employee has more choice in how he or she chooses to spend the money. The benefit to the employer is that if the employees are behaving like smart shoppers to get more for that amount, their premiums might not increase as rapidly.

Tips for Using Medical Savings Accounts (MSAs)

Understand the rules and the details of the rules as they apply to timing and use of the funds.

Timing is everything with medical savings accounts. For example, if you need a new pair of glasses and they're covered by the plan, you might want to buy them near the end of the coverage period to make sure you use up what is available in your medical savings account before the end of the plan period. Early in the period's year, you might not put through claims for certain items in case an emergency requiring expensive drugs or care occurs later.

Claiming under Private Insurance Plans

It is important to understand your benefits plan or plans so that you don't leave a lot of money on the table that could be in your pocket. You may even avoid getting important health care services for you and your family because you don't understand how the benefit plan can support you financially.

Many Canadians fail to successfully claim their full entitlement under these benefits plans because they don't really know the rules of their plan or some of the basic tips to maximizing it. They also don't understand how to expedite the process of making a claim.

Practical experience has taught us that insurance companies are pretty quick to reject claims or return them *sans* cheque if any little piece of information is missing or if their procedures have not been followed. Basic protocols exist within the insurance industry for handling claims, and there are specific things that your insurance company requires. These tend to be standard fare. One common requirement is this: All insurance companies need original, official receipts, not credit card receipts, for items that they have agreed to cover. Another is that the application must be signed and dated by the insured (or the person covered even if the claim is for a family member). All family members must be listed with the insurance company when you become insured or their claims will not be accepted.

Let's just review the basics of making a claim:

- Ascertain that your plan covers the medication, service, or equipment you are claiming for. You can find this information by checking your plan guide or contacting your insurance company. If you are in an employer-sponsored program, your director of human resources might know the answer or be able to find out for you.

- Photocopy or scan into your computer every piece of paper you are sending to the insurance company. Don't forget the backs of forms, too.
- Before stuffing all the bits of paper in the envelope, review all the forms you have had to fill out (or have your spouse or someone else take a look at them). A fresh eye can catch little boxes you've forgotten to tick or vital information you haven't filled in. Check off that you've included all the documentation asked for.
- Make a note to yourself of the day you posted the package.

Tip

Caveat! Operate on the principle that whatever you send to an insurance company is never returned. Make copies of everything before you send your package off. You will need to copy each of the receipts you are submitting.

Coordinating Two Benefits Plans

When there are two benefits plans in a family, who claims what? In the case of married or common-law couples, each spouse must claim his or her personal health care and dental care expenses with his or her own insurance company first. What many people don't realize is that the portion not paid by the first spouse's insurance company can then be submitted to the other spouse's plan. Yes, you can do that! But you need to claim on both plans to get your full benefit. How you do it will be explained below. This is pretty straightforward. But it gets more complicated when children's claims are involved.

Tips

- Assess your family situation before deciding whether to have two health plans in your household.
- If you have two plans, remember to claim the difference on your partner's plan!

Coordinating Benefits for Children under Two Plans

If both spouses have benefits plans that include family coverage, the parent whose birthday comes first (month and day) will submit the child's claim through his or her insurance company first. He or she will be considered the "primary claimant" and this will be the "primary claim." Primary claims must include the original receipt for the service or medicine as well as a properly filled out claim form.

The insurance company will then provide the primary claimant with a reimbursement cheque and an Explanation of Benefits (EOB) statement. This is the official document that outlines how much you claimed and how much you were reimbursed. If there is a difference, the EOB will explain why you didn't receive the full amount. The other parent (the secondary claimant) then can submit to his or her insurance company the primary claimant's EOB statement from the spouse's insurance company. The second claim usually makes up the difference.

Here's a practical example of how this works: If Emily's birthday is July 1 and her husband Peter's birthday is June 15, then Peter would be the first claimant (regardless of the year in which they were born). Peter would submit a receipt, let's say for $100, for his child's medicine to his insurance company. If his insurance company doesn't charge a deductible but reimburses only 80 percent of eligible claims, Peter would get back $80 and an EOB statement. Emily, the second claimant, will file the second claim with her insurance company and her husband's EOB statement. Her insurance company would also cover only 80 percent of the eligible amount of the medication, but since Peter's company has paid out that amount already, the second insurance company will reimburse enough to make up the full cost. Obviously, the second company will not reimburse what has already been reimbursed by Peter's insurance company. Emily will get back $20. In short, she will get back 100 percent of the amount not covered by Peter's insurance company. This is because insurance companies reimburse a certain percentage (in her case 80 percent) of the total cost of the drug and not 80 percent of the outstanding amount being claimed. Many people get confused here. The cost to Emily and Peter will be zero, but only if they know how to properly submit their two claims.

Tip

Q: My husband has a great benefits plan through his work—they reimburse 100 percent on eligible drugs and there is no deductible! I am starting a new job. Should I bother to get family benefits?

A: We don't believe in overinsuring, but too many times this question is answered without the proper assessment being done. Many times it makes sense to have two plans. For example, when it comes to things like orthodontics, there is power in numbers—that is, the number of plans your family can access for the purpose of reimbursement. Also, as seen above, when your plan doesn't cover everything it is often good to be able to claim on another plan. Review your situation, the age of your children, and other factors such as family medical history, then make an informed decision. Here are some things to consider:

- Are my kids going to need orthodontic work soon?
- Are my family's prescription drug costs or medical costs high in relation to how much I would pay on premiums to maintain this plan? (If you are paying a $300-per-month premium out of your own pocket or paycheque, and your family's needs aren't great, it may not be worth it.)
- What other benefits do I get that I should keep, like life insurance or disability?

Find out from your insurance company what you need to do the first time you claim this way to ensure that the coordination of benefits is recorded properly—who is the first claimant and what the terms of that person's insurance are. If you don't submit properly the first time, the two insurance companies will need to contact each other for verification. This could take a while and, not surprisingly, usually does. Verify that all you need to submit is the other person's EOB without photocopied receipts.

When this process has been gone through the first time, the insurance companies log which parent is the secondary claimant (or the primary) with regard to their kids' claims. After this is established, claims go more smoothly.

Coordination of Benefits for Orthodontics

Orthodontic treatment to straighten your son's or daughter's teeth can easily cost between $3000 and $5000—this is a big-ticket item for most families. Insurers will typically offer only up to 50 percent coverage on eligible orthodontic expenses up to a certain amount—often capped at $2000 or so per child. If both parents have coverage, they can submit using the procedure of primary and secondary claim described above. If both parents are eligible for 50 percent of the total amount paid, between them they will recoup the entire expense they paid up to the capped limit.

As an example, if your child's orthodontic expenses were to be $4000, with only one family plan capped at $2000, your family would be able to get back half of the cost of the orthodontics, or $2000. With two plans each reimbursing you $2000, you would be reimbursed for the full amount.

God is in the details when it comes to insurance plans. You must understand the specifics of how much (in percentage) the insurance company will reimburse, on what items, and up to what amount (in dollars) before you can properly assess the relative risk of using some of that coverage.

There is no one-size-fits-all rule when it comes to deciding whether to put another policy in place or just use your spouse's plan. Look at it this way: If you have a family of five kids who all have major overbites, the amount your employer will deduct on your pay for your portion of the benefit premium might be worth it.

Tips

If you and your spouse have dental coverage, make the dentist aware of both plans and their details. You may have coverage for a certain procedure under a spouse's benefit plan that you are unaware of. If your plan doesn't cover your dental work, it may be that your spouse's will cover it.

Find out exactly what documents your insurance company needs before you make the first claim for orthodontic treatment. Often they will require a signed contract for the services and proof from the dentist that the service was paid in full. Note that credit card receipts or statements will not qualify as proof.

Big tip regarding orthodontics! Often it is very easy for the first claimant to get back 50 percent of the expense, but the second claimant has trouble when the insurance company decides to reimburse 50 percent of the 50 percent remaining to be paid rather than 50 percent of the total cost. If your plan says you are entitled to 50 percent of the cost of orthodontic treatment up to a certain amount, make sure both you and your spouse or partner each get back 50 percent of the entire bill. Hold the insurer's feet to the fire!

Coordination of Benefits in a Divorce

What do you do when you and your spouse are separated or divorced? Which parent's benefit plan covers the child or children?

If both parents have an employer-sponsored plan, both should continue to maintain family health insurance coverage to support the child's needs, regardless of where he or she resides. Although courts and legal documents don't comment on how the coordination of benefits works, insurance companies have protocols in place to deal with these situations.

Most people don't know the rules of the game, but insurance companies have a policy on such a situation. Manulife Financial explains the protocol that insurance companies follow:

> The order of submission for coordination of benefits, in a case where the parents are divorced (separated), is as follows:
>
> 1. The plan of the parent with custody of the child, then
> 2. The plan of the spouse of the parent with custody of the child (new spouse), then
> 3. The plan of the parent not having custody of the child, then
> 4. The plan of the spouse of the parent without custody of the child (new spouse).

Note that just as the legal system may not be the authority on the intricacies of benefits protocols, insurance companies don't use the correct terminology when they talk about custody. For the insurance profession the parent who has custody is the one with whom the child resides. So if you are in a joint-custody arrangement but the children live most of the time with you, you are the first claimant according to the insurance industry. They should change the wording from the "parent with custody" to "the parent with whom the children reside." Also, note that "spouse" nowadays includes "common-law partner" as defined under the law and as recognized by most insurance companies.

The spirit of the rule, however, is logical. If a child resides with one parent, usually it is this parent who takes the child to the doctor, dentist, or orthodontist more often and often pays for the expenses up front. Therefore it is this parent who should make the first claim. The first-claimant parent will then submit the Explanation of Benefit to the second-claimant parent, who will claim any amount that has not been reimbursed. The money that the second claimant receives should be returned to the parent who paid the whole bill out of pocket.

In divorces, the standard clause in most settlements (where both parents have group dental and extended health and drug plans through their respective employers) is all about safeguarding general principles to ensure that no one parent will be on the hook for out-of-pocket expenses related to health and dental.

When legal divorce agreements are dealing with insurance provisions, they tend to be worded something like the following:

> The husband and the wife are each presently covered by benefit plans. They will both continue this coverage for the children, so long as the children (or any of them) remain children as defined in the Child Support Guidelines.
>
> Where one party ("the payer") is obliged to pay a fee directly to a dentist, hospital, health care facility or druggist in relation to any services which are covered in all or in part by the plans referred to herein, the other party will immediately endorse over to the payer any cheque received from the plan or plans in reimbursement of all or part of the services for which the payer has paid directly.
>
> The husband and wife will share equally any health care or treatment expenses which are not covered by insurance, including non-insured services and orthodontic treatment.

Good legal agreements support the provision that both parents have coverage for the children so that if one plan doesn't cover a particular need, there is another that possibly does. Of course, everything in a divorce situation is open to negotiation.

The second and third paragraphs are fairly self-explanatory but are not always included in legal agreements. If one parent pays directly for expenses, and the other makes the claim on his or her insurance, the payer is entitled to get back the amount reimbursed by the insurance company. Where there is an out-of-pocket difference, both parents will share in the portion of out-of-pocket expenses that the plans do not cover.

If your divorce settlement doesn't put these insurance provisions in writing, it should. Health care costs can be enormous and many plans don't cover 100 percent of them. Usually child support payments are adjusted on a yearly basis according to income. This annual event may provide a good opportunity to include these provisions if they are missing from your agreement.

Here is another good clause that divorce agreements don't necessarily include but should. It deals with coordination of benefits and ensures that each party will act in good faith by exchanging the documents that the other may require to claim on his or her plan:

> The parties agree to immediately exchange any documentation of payment, which includes the amounts paid by the insurance company to the first claimant, in order to maximize the amounts they can receive from their respective insurance companies.

Remember the importance of having the second claimant submit the Explanation of Benefits from the first claimant? Well, guess what? Insurance companies don't actually care whether the situation between your ex and you is amicable or not. *They will not overpay a claim*, and they therefore will need the Explanation of Benefits from your ex-spouse's insurance company. The only way they will know that they are not overpaying a claim is if the second claimant can produce documentation from the first insurance company saying exactly what the claim was and how much they paid out.

Of course, when the first claimant is the one who paid out of pocket, it is in his or her best interest to provide the other parent with the Explanation of Benefits so that the first claimant can be reimbursed all the money he or she paid. So why do you need this clause? The fact is that for things like orthodontics, where the upfront costs are big, many dentists will suggest that each parent pay 50 percent. They both can submit. The problem is that insurance companies still need to coordinate benefits the same way it is explained under "Coordination of Benefits for Orthodontics." So if the first claimant decides to be nasty, he or she can get the original documents, claim the full amount (as is right), get his or her 50 percent back, and not bother providing all necessary documentation (including the EOB statement) to the second claimant. The second claimant is left with a big expense and no paperwork to get reimbursed for his or her 50 percent of the total cost.

These clauses are fair and self-evident. Unfortunately, divorce situations often lead to parties adopting the unreasonable attitude of "It's not in the agreement, so I don't have to do it." With the cost of legal advice so high these days, it often isn't worth taking legal action to recuperate what you've paid. If your separation or divorce agreement includes these clauses and the other person is in breach of this agreement, he or she may be ordered by a court to pay what is owed plus any legal expenses you incur trying to rectify the situation. This alone is usually enough to make certain everyone plays by the rules. If these things are not in your agreement, get them in there!

Tip

The same tips apply in divorce situations as in the coordination of benefits. The only addition here is to ensure that all the seemingly self-evident clauses are put into your agreement.

Prescription Drugs

Private plans usually cover, on some basis, a portion of drug costs. While very few plans cover the full costs, most of them will have a formula whereby they cover something like 75 or 80 percent of the costs of drugs. Some plans will provide you with a plastic benefit card that you can present at the retail pharmacy when you get a prescription filled. The pharmacist will swipe your card and, in many cases, bill directly to the company their portion, leaving you to pay the balance, which is usually a portion of the dispensing fee (depending how much your plan covers). Otherwise, you need to collect your original receipts and file the claim by filling out the forms and mailing them in as we explained above.

The drug component of your benefits plan can prove to be important, particularly if you are on high-cost maintenance drugs, drugs that you may need to take for the rest of your life. It is not unusual for an individual in his or her 50s or 60s to incur a cost of $60 to $70 per month for each maintenance drug. Many Canadians are spending in excess of $100 or even $200 a month for a variety of medications from which they are deriving benefit. Payment for these medications can be quite a burden.

Tip

Often benefits plans will pay different portions of the dispensing fee and the drug costs. It might be in your interest to shop for a pharmacy that combines convenience—you don't want to drive 20 kilometres to save $2 of a dispensing fee—with a lower dispensing fee or no fee at all.

If you don't have a plastic card that automatically debits the insurance company and you must pay up front and then claim after, make sure you have a file where you can amass your pharmacy receipts! Carelessness in misplacing these receipts means Canadians fail to claim millions of dollars every year in benefits.

Dental

Another area of plans is dental care and here you need to work very closely with your dentist. Plan coverage is often complicated. In the case of routine cleanings, generally you pay the dentist, who files an electronic claim with the insurance company on your behalf. You then receive a cheque from the insurance company for its portion of the payment. Most Canadian dentists now accept major credit cards, a service that facilitates transactions. In the case of major dental work, often a dentist will send an estimate or quote to the insurance company so that it can determine in advance what portion, if any, of the work being done will be covered.

An extreme example came from a friend of Michael's, who needed a great deal of restorative dental work, including very expensive dental implants, shortly before he retired from the company where he'd worked for 14 years. He was not sure what was covered by his policy, so he took the dental plan, the actual document, to his dentist, who said, "Whoopee! A gold mine!" It turned out that in this particular instance, the company plan would pay 100 percent of the costs of dental implants. Michael's friend had what can only be described as a total dental makeover, including a number of dental implants. The total bill was nearly $40,000. The total cost to the friend was $0. The dentist was able to bill the entire procedure to the insurance company. We want to emphasize that this was an extreme case, with extensive and expensive restorative work and an unbelievably good dental plan. But it's a cautionary tale: Get to know the details of your insurance plan.

Dental plans usually will pay only up to a certain amount as recommended by the General Practitioner Dental Association Fee Guide of your province. If your dentist chooses to charge more—and he or she is absolutely allowed to do so—your plan probably won't cover the difference.

Tips

If cost is important to you, make sure you have a dentist who charges within the fee schedule that your plan reimburses. Find out what your plan uses as the recommended guide and take that to your dentist. Ask your dentist if he or she charges more for the service.

Make sure you know how many procedures—cleanings, scalings, etc.—you can have done in a year and how many weeks or months need to pass between each. Make your dentist aware of this restriction. If you need something done immediately but your plan will cover it only if you wait another few days, a dentist is sometimes willing to help by changing the schedule date of the service provided.

Medical Devices

This is another area in which it's up to you to find out what is covered. There are many different types of medical devices, and policies vary greatly on what they cover. Many of these devices are listed in a chart in Chapter 10, "Navigating Health Care for Seniors."

A medical device that is often covered is foot orthotics. Many workers, particularly workers who spend a great deal of time on their feet, develop soreness that could be alleviated with the use of foot orthotics (an insert that goes in your shoe, conforms to your foot, and spreads the pressure in a way that alleviates both foot pain and, in many cases, back pain). Orthotics can be expensive, running to $200 or $300 a pair. However, many benefits plans for unionized workers, who spend a lot time on their feet, such as teachers and nurses, include coverage for orthotics. So if you are a teacher or a nurse, or an auto worker in an assembly plant with foot or back pain, there are two things you can do for yourself. First, see a registered foot doctor, a podiatrist, or other doctor specializing in problems of the foot, and second, check your benefits plan to see if you are covered for orthotics. Most plans provide for a replacement every two years, so even if you have orthotics, you might want to get a new pair when you're eligible. This way you aren't moving them from one pair of shoes to the other and they will remain effective and fresh for longer.

Some years ago, Francesca had a terrible lower back pain and was put on strong anti-inflammatory medications that cost a fortune (and did nothing to help the pain). She was having to miss work because she could barely walk. When she was well enough to return to work, she bought an Obus Forme backrest support for her chair, and it helped a great deal. The insurance company wouldn't cover the cost of the device, so Francesca called a claims broker (the representative you complain to when your claim isn't honoured) and fought like hell. Her argument was simple: She sat a great deal on a lousy chair while at work. That is what brought on the problem. The insurance company could pay for an ergonomic chair, cover her short-term disability (which she almost applied for), or continue to pick up the bill for her meds. All options over time would prove to be much more expensive than the Obus Forme. The company covered the device.

Allied Health Professionals

Allied health professionals include chiropractors, massage therapists, optometrists, and dietitians, among others. For you to claim expenses for visits to any type of allied health professional, he or she must provide you with an invoice marked "Paid" and his or her registered practitioner number. Many plans have provisions to

Tips

Check with your insurance company to find out what types of allied health professionals are covered. And be prepared to fight for the grey areas.

If you are having a baby and have secured the assistance of a doula who is also a registered nurse, ask her to give you an invoice for services with her registered nursing number on it. You usually cannot be reimbursed for doula services on standard benefits plans, but you can be reimbursed for services provided by a registered nurse. Getting reimbursed by a benefits plan is worth a great deal more to you than being able to make a claim for medical expenses on your income tax, as you will see in the next chapter, "Claiming Medical Expenses on Your Tax Return."

cover a fixed number of visits per year. In addition, massage therapists need to have a practice registration number to show they are registered with their professional governing body. Not everyone giving you a massage will be reimbursed. They need to be a professional massage therapist and will need a registration number to prove it.

Critical Illness Insurance

The decision about whether to buy critical illness insurance is not an easy one to make. First, you need to know which illnesses are considered critical. Critical illnesses usually include stroke, heart disease, cancer, kidney failure, and multiple sclerosis, among others. The illnesses and maximum benefit depend on the insurance company and should be spelled out clearly in your documents. You should be aware that critical illness insurance does not typically cover you when your illness is HIV. The insurance is paid out only if your diagnosis and the severity of your case meet the criteria set out in the policy. So you must be mindful of what you are signing up for.

If you become ill with one of the diseases or conditions specified in your insurance agreement, the insurance is paid in a lump sum when you notify your insurer that you are ill. You will need to ask the insurance company what they need in the way of documentation, since it differs from company to company. You can use the money for anything you want: access to medical expertise around the world, alternative therapies, medications that the government will not cover, household help (nannies to take care of your kids while you recover from treatment, housekeepers, cook), vacations, clothing, etc. Depending on the plan you choose, the lump sum can be between $50,000 and $2,000,000.

You will not need to provide receipts. You will not need to have reported income in order to get the benefit (as is the case with disability insurance). Also, if you return to work, you can still keep the critical illness insurance money—you do not have to repay it.

The main criterion used to determine eligibility for payment is whether you have been diagnosed by a medical professional with a critical illness as defined by your plan. Typically, you will need to have survived the critical illness for a period that is set out in your plan (usually 30 days). If this seems too good to be true, that is because we haven't discussed costs yet.

This type of insurance is not cheap. Premiums vary depending on the insurance company and also on your age and other health factors. Premiums can range from $20 to $30 per month for a 35- to 40-year-old healthy non-smoker. But this will buy only about $100,000 worth of insurance. You can imagine how much it might cost to purchase $2,000,000 worth. Still, it is a great idea if you can afford it. In some sense, it is like a forced savings plan. You put money into the plan every month and if you are diagnosed with a critical illness, it pays out. Of course, if you never develop a critical illness you lose your money—however, most of us will at some point have a critical illness.

Another thing to keep in mind: Currently this insurance is treated as a life insurance payout for tax purposes. This means that the money you receive is tax free. However, tax regulations, as well as types of critical illness insurance, are changing all the time, so when you're investigating this type of insurance, be sure to check the tax implications.

> **Tip**
>
> Make sure your family members are informed of specialized insurance you have purchased and know where the relevant documents are. If you become incapacitated, they will be able to ensure that you receive the benefits you have been paying for.

Long-term Care Insurance

Another relatively new product is long-term care insurance, which is provided in Canada only by a handful of insurers. In fact, it is so new that the insurance companies offering this product will guarantee the premiums for only about five years, after which they reserve the right to increase the cost if they find it isn't feasible to continue offering the product at previous rates. Their ability to hold the premium at the same cost will depend on sales volume and also on claims made, information that is currently almost nonexistent.

In Chapter 10, "Navigating Health Care for Seniors," we discuss the implications of our aging population. Health Canada reports that seniors over age 65 are the fastest-growing population group in the country. We are also living longer. These two things mean that affordable government-funded home care may be limited in scope. It also means that wait times are often very long to get into good government-funded nursing home facilities. We also talk about some of the costs associated with private care. It is important to note that some younger people also require long-term care at home or in an institution. This type of insurance helps pay the cost of long-term care whether it is accommodation in a private facility or professional care in your own home.

Long-term care plans can be purchased after the age of 30. These plans offer a number of choices, including the length of the benefit period and the amount of the benefit, which of course will be reflected in the premium you pay; you can apply for a monthly benefit from $300 to $9000 per month. The average long-term care facility today costs about $2000 to $3000 per month. Some insurers will require receipts before they pay out the benefit; others will not.

You qualify to receive your long-term care benefit when you become unable to perform two activities of daily living—for example, feeding and bathing—or you lose key functions, such as cognitive ability. Before receiving benefits, you will need to fulfill an "elimination period," which means that you will not receive any money during that time. It will be important to check how your insurance company defines an elimination period. Sometimes it will be calculated in calendar days from the time you are diagnosed. Other times, they will include only the number of days in which you actually get into a long-term care facility or have received the services of home care.

The tax consequences for long-term care insurance are not clear. It may get treated like the old Survivors' Income Benefit (which was subject to being taxed). Again, you really need to talk to your accountant and factor his or her answers into your decisions.

Medicare Eligibility

What happens if you move from one province to another? Whose medicare plan are you covered under?

You will be covered under your old province's plan until you fulfill the eligibility requirement—which is usually a 90-day period. For example, if you move from Manitoba to Ontario, for your first 90 days in Ontario you would still be covered by the Manitoba health insurance plan before Ontario's plan would kick in. This is in part to allow time to obtain a new health card. *It is important to keep your health card from your original province until you receive your new card.* If you are moving back to Canada from abroad, rules vary, but generally 90 days is the standard waiting time before you are covered under your province or territory's plan. In British Columbia, it is three months, but the first part-month is counted as a full month, so your eligibility waiting period might be somewhat less than 90 days. Websites for provincial and territorial health ministries will inform you about their eligibility requirements and how to apply for a new health card.

Generally, when you leave your province or territory to travel inside Canada, you're covered by medicare. Reciprocal arrangements among provinces under the portability provisions of the Canada Health Act have ensured this coverage for all Canadians. For most Canadians travelling to another province, obtaining health care is as simple as producing your provincial or territorial health card to allow the health facility in the other province to bill the charge back to your home province. The only exception to this rule is that some Quebec residents have encountered difficulties in different parts of the country because rate structures and timing of payments by the Quebec government's Régis seem to lag compared to other parts of the country. In general, when you are travelling in Canada you needn't worry about supplementary health insurance.

Out-of-Country Insurance

The only thing worse than being sick away from home is being seriously ill away from home with no medical coverage. When you travel outside Canada, it is essential that you maintain health insurance coverage. The first step in this process is to understand what will be covered by medicare when you are outside your province, your territory, or Canada. The second step is to find out what additional coverage you may have and not even know about under your existing employer or private plans. Many employer plans provide for some out-of-country coverage. Even credit cards may provide some out-of-country or travel insurance medical coverage, but it's important to understand the terms and conditions—for example, you might have to pay for the trip with a particular card to activate the medical coverage. It is also possible, particularly for short trips, to buy relatively inexpensive insurance.

If you are planning a longer time out of the country, you should check carefully how this can affect your eligibility for continuing coverage by medicare. Your provincial health insurance coverage will lapse if you are out of the country for a certain period of time—check with your province's ministry of health.

The moment you step outside Canada you are well advised to have travel medical insurance. Much of the

Tip

Your travel agent, bank, or doctor can advise you about options for supplementary insurance. Some credit card companies offer their holders health and travel insurance. Coverage may not be automatically included or may not on its own be adequate. You may be required to pay an additional premium for travel coverage and you may have to pay for your travel arrangements using that card to initiate the coverage. Check the conditions, limitations, and requirements before you leave.

advice that follows is based on recommendations from the Government of Canada:

- Before leaving Canada, buy supplementary medical insurance. Your provincial health plan may not cover costs incurred if you become sick or injured while abroad. For example, the Government of Saskatchewan says that if the cost of treatment services outside Canada is higher than what Saskatchewan reimburses, residents are required to pay the difference between the amount charged and what the provincial health plan pays.
- Keep proof of insurance coverage with your other travel documents and give a copy to someone at home.
- Do not rely on your provincial health plan to cover costs if you get sick or are injured while abroad. At best, your health plan will cover only a portion of the bill. It is your responsibility to obtain and understand the terms of your supplementary travel insurance policy.
- With all insurance policies, examine the details. For travel insurance you will want to know whether there is an emergency hotline available 24 hours a day; how a foreign hospital will be reimbursed—up front by you or later by your insurance company; whether medical evacuation is covered and a medical escort will accompany you; whether pre-existing conditions are covered; what happens if you die abroad.

- Here are some details to ask about: Does the insurer have an in-house, worldwide emergency hotline you can call if you are in trouble? Does it operate 24 hours a day, seven days a week? Are the operators multilingual? Are there nurses or physicians on staff? You can decide how important each of these is to you.
- You will want to know how the bills are to be paid. Does the insurer pay foreign hospital and related medical costs? Are you expected to pay on the spot or will the insurer pay the hospital immediately? Will the plan allow for cash advances if a doctor or hospital requires immediate payment?
- Get a detailed invoice from the doctor or hospital before you leave the country. Submit original receipts for medical services or prescriptions received abroad. Most insurance companies will not accept copies or faxes. Keep a copy of the submitted documents for your files.
- Some insurers provide for medical evacuation to Canada or the nearest location with appropriate medical care. They may also pay for a medical escort (doctor or nurse) to accompany you during evacuation. This service can cost as much as $100,000 if it is not included.
- If you have a pre-existing medical condition, clarify whether this is covered. Get an agreement in writing from your insurer that you are covered for such conditions. You could find your claim considered null and void if you have a pre-existing condition clause.

- If you're pregnant, it will be important to know if the plan covers premature births and related neonatal care.
- If you were to die abroad, would the plan pay for the preparation and return of your remains to Canada? Otherwise, this service can cost as much as $10,000.
- If you are abroad for an extended period of time, your provincial health insurance plan will become invalid. The period varies by province. You are advised to buy personal medical insurance if you will be living outside Canada for an extended period.

Tip

Make sure you have coverage for a partial-day out-of-country shopping trip! Check your insurance policies and buy short-term coverage, if necessary. Many accidents happen on these short excursions.

Do some homework on this topic by going to www.ontarioinsurance.com. Go to the Consumer Brochures section and scroll down to the heading "Life and Health Insurance" to download a brochure called *Shopping for Travel Medical Insurance*, published by the Financial Services Commission of Ontario. This guide covers many of the important topics we've noted. You can also go direct to people selling insurance. Many provinces have Blue Cross organizations, which sell supplementary insurance that adds to your government coverage. Some provincial governments provide modest coverage outside

Canada, but it is generally insufficient to the task that you may face in any urgent situation. In addition to Blue Cross, a number of insurance companies, including Manulife Financial, Great West Life, and Sun Life, provide out-of-country insurance.

Applying for personal insurance of any type doesn't guarantee that you will be successful in getting the coverage you need. Obviously, insurance companies make money on healthy clients, not the unhealthy clients. And, unless you happen to be 35 and very healthy, applying for coverage is a longer process than you might expect. You will probably be asked a number of questions and perhaps be subjected to a visit by a nurse who will take blood and urine samples and run a number of other tests as well. This is how insurance companies can properly assess the potential risk they carry in offering you insurance.

Likewise, you need to check the insurance company's offering. For most of us who have some illness or condition, applying for health insurance is unlikely to be a quick task. If it is, chances are the plan you are getting will not be such a great deal. You will almost certainly be overlooking the details of what you're buying. With all private health insurance plans, the devil is in the details. Ask lots of questions. Make sure you either meet in person or connect by phone with a representative. Either way, take notes! Make sure you know exactly what you are buying.

If you have to fight with an insurance company over a grey area, remember that they are in business to make money—certainly not to lose money. The most compelling argument is a cost benefit argument. In short, if you pay for this condition, I won't be claiming for that condition. "That condition" must be shown to be more expensive than "this condition."

RESOURCE GUIDE

BOOKS

The Insurance Book: What Canadians Really Need to Know Before Buying Insurance. Sally Praskey and Helena Moncrieff (Toronto: Prentice Hall, 1999).

This excellent book, endorsed by the Consumers Council of Canada, will provide you with a detailed guide to private insurance of all kinds. However, it also covers health insurance, including what private plans cover, whether you need disability insurance, and what to do if you disagree with the insurance company's decision about your claim. A must-read for Canadians interested in understanding insurance plans from a practical point of view.

ORGANIZATIONS AND ASSOCIATIONS

Insurance-Canada.ca
www.insurance-canada.ca

While there are numerous insurance company sites, Insurance-Canada.ca is the best resource we have come across to help navigate all types of insurance for Canadian consumers. It provides concise and easy-to-understand overviews of the types of insurance available and how they work, as well as tips and links to the companies that provide these products.

GOVERNMENT PROGRAMS

Service Canada
www.canadabenefits.gc.ca
Use this excellent website to locate all the government drug programs in your province. First, access the website homepage. Do not click on anything under the first column, labelled "I am" (a parent, a senior, a student). Instead click "Health Concerns," under the column entitled "Life Events."

You will then see a map of Canada. Click on your province or territory.

The next page will allow you to click on one of three themes:

- Health and Dental Care: This will give you links and listings for government-sponsored programs related to assistive devices for you or your children and other special programs.
- Mental Health Counseling and Addictions: This will help you access government programs that provide you with benefits in these areas.

- Prescription Drug Coverage: This will provide you with what your government offers in drug coverage and catastrophic drug coverage.

Public Health Agency of Canada
www.travelhealth.gc.ca
The Travel Medicine Program (TMP) is responsible for providing the following travel health information for persons travelling outside Canada:

- Current information on international disease outbreaks
- Immunization recommendations for international travel
- General health advice for international travellers
- Disease-specific treatment and prevention guidelines

Information can be accessed 24 hours a day through the Internet at the address above. This information has been specifically designed for persons planning to travel internationally and for travel medicine professionals who provide counsel to international travellers.

SIX

Claiming Medical Expenses on Your Tax Return

Are you claiming every medical expense that you are eligible to claim on your income taxes? For many of us, the answer is "Probably not."

The Canadian Institute for Health Information (CIHI) reports that, on average, Canadians spend about $17 billion on out-of-pocket medical expenses annually. At the same time, the Canada Revenue Agency (CRA) reported that in 2000 the government paid out about half a billion dollars on medical expense claims. The CRA is projecting that by 2007 it will pay almost a billion dollars. This jump, according to the CRA, is largely the result of a growth in medical spending by Canadians and also because the government has expanded the list of medical expenses that can be claimed. Still, it is reasonable to believe that Canadians are leaving money on the table.

It is true that what you can and cannot declare is a bit of a moving target. The good news is that the target seems to be moving in the right direction for the taxpayer. Over the last few years (from about 2004 to the present), each federal budget has added items or expanded what can be claimed as a medical expense. Still, there are many medical expenses that cannot be claimed. And understanding this complicated policy area is challenging.

A number of court decisions have interpreted which medical claims will and will not be allowed, and this will continue. That these questions have to be resolved in court is a testament to the fact that there are many grey areas, some more grey than others. However, there are a few clear no-nos that have evolved when it comes to claiming medical expenses. Let's begin at what is *not* claimable. When it comes to legitimate medical expenses, only a relatively few are not allowed.

What Is *Not* Claimable

Any expense that has already been reimbursed either by a government-sponsored health plan or by your employer's or your own private health plan cannot be claimed on your personal taxes. Sensibly, you cannot be paid twice! This means you cannot claim any medical expense for which you are entitled to be reimbursed but for which you paid. For example, you forget your medicare card when you go for an X-ray; you are covered for this service under your provincial health plan but, in the absence of a medicare card, the lab charges you. You cannot claim this expense on your income tax, because it is up to you to provide your medicare card. After the fact you may provide your medicare card and the charges will be reversed within a certain time period, but you may not claim charges on your income tax in these cases.

The same is true if you have an employer drug plan and you don't claim your reimbursement on that plan. You cannot claim as a medical expense on your income tax anything for which you are entitled to be reimbursed on any health plan (public, employer, or private) that you have. In any case, claiming medical expenses on your income tax is never as beneficial as getting reimbursement in whole or in part from your health insurance plan.

Generally, non-prescription medicines and devices are not claimable, though there are exceptions to this rule, as we will see.

Vitamins and supplements are not claimable unless they have been prescribed by a physician and have been purchased in a pharmacy and dispensed and recorded by the pharmacist.

You cannot claim as a medical expense a home renovation or improvement that would either

- raise the value of your home or

- be typically undertaken by people who are not afflicted with a similar impairment.

For example, if you use a wheelchair and need to put an elevator in your home, that would be acceptable. If you decide to put in an outdoor Jacuzzi for your bad back, that will be a much tougher sell to the CRA. Francesca's accountant, Glenn Lott, had a case of a person who legitimately needed a hot tub to treat a health affliction. The person had an official document from his doctor that clearly stated that the hot tub was necessary for his afflictions. Some $12,000 later the hot tub was installed, and the person claimed the hot tub on his next tax return. The result? The CRA asked to see all the receipts. And, though they did not allow him to claim the cost of the hot tub, they did allow the $2000 expense to install it. It would seem that sometimes there are some grey areas from which you can benefit!

You cannot claim premiums paid by you under any provincial or territorial government medical or hospitalization plans, but you can claim premiums if they are for private insurance and have been paid by you, not your employer.

Now let's look at how the different kinds of medical expenses are categorized.

Categories of Medical Expenses

When declaring medical expenses, you must understand that some qualify as credits, some as refunds, and some as deductions. There are important differences between these categories.

Most medical expenses (listed below) are *not* deductions but rather tax credits. What does that mean and why is it important to you?

Tax Deductions

A *tax deduction* is something that reduces the income on which taxes are calculated. The tax saving you get is dependent on your personal income tax rate. The higher your tax bracket, the greater is the benefit of the deduction. If you are in a 46 percent tax bracket, for example, you will get back 46 cents on every dollar spent on eligible tax-deductible items. If you overpaid taxes (once the deductions are calculated), you will be refunded the amount of taxes you overpaid. If you don't pay taxes, the deduction will be of no benefit.

Tax Credits

Tax credits, like deductions, are applied against the tax you owe or the tax you paid. However, unlike tax deductions, tax credits are not based on your personal income tax rate. They are based on the lowest federal tax rate, which was 15 percent in 2005, 15.25 percent in 2006, and 15.50 percent in 2007, combined with your lowest provincial tax rate. So if you are earning a high income, you will not get your tax rate back. This means that what you get back will have nothing to do with the percentage of tax you pay. People in a high income bracket will get back only around 16 percent of the amount that is eligible for the credit. As we will see, the amount upon which the 16 percent is calculated is not the total of all your bills but a percentage of them.

Medical Tax Credits

As explained, the *medical tax credit* is one of the credits in which the less you earn the greater the benefit, and vice versa. Here is how the calculation works: All your medical expenses are added together. This number is then reduced by 3 percent of your net income or $1844, whichever is less. Everyone, regardless of income, would get a tax credit of approximately 16 percent of the rest. Since the amount you need to subtract from your expenses is either 3 percent of net income or $1844, it is obvious that the lower your income, the less you will deduct from your expenses. If you earn $10,000 per year, you will subtract only $300 whereas a person who earns $70,000 will subtract the entire $1844. After that, everyone gets around a 16 percent tax credit regardless of earnings. That is why generally anything that falls into this category is best claimed by the lower-income earner. However, if both family earners have very high incomes, it would be beneficial for the higher-income earner to claim this credit—people in a very high income bracket have to pay surtaxes and this credit could reduce the surtax.

Below is an example of the calculation for a person with a net income of $40,000:

Eligible medical expenses – $5000 in 12 months
Minus 3% of net income – $1200
Amount – $4800
Tax credit will be around 16% of $4800 = $768

This person would receive a tax credit of $768. Had medical expenses been a tax deduction, this person would have received a tax benefit of approximately 22 percent plus the corresponding provincial tax rate of the medical expense, based on his tax rate.

Medical Supplemental "Refund" (or Rebate)

The term medical supplemental "refund" is not really a very accurate way of describing this tax break. A "refund" implies that money is given back to you for what you have paid or what you owe. However, the medical supplemental "refund" is really much more of a rebate because, if you meet the requirement, it doesn't matter whether you have paid taxes, owe taxes or not. You will get it. So we will refer to this as a rebate. Rebates have different calculations (some take into account your income, others do not). There is usually a limit to how much of a rebate the government is ready to pay out. The big difference between a rebate and a credit or deduction is that if you don't owe any tax, you *will still* get the rebate. If you do owe tax, your rebate will be offset against what you owe.

Who Claims What and How

Not only do you have to know how to navigate the health system, it's advantageous to know how to navigate the income tax system! Even if you have someone else do your taxes, you should understand the types of medical expenses categories we described above, as well as what can be claimed and by whom. After all, you are the one giving the information and bits of paper to your tax preparer—you don't want to miss anything that will be beneficial to you. One important thing to remember is that besides declaring medical expenses for yourself, you can declare expenses for dependants as well. However, the relationship these people have to you makes a difference to where you can declare these things on your tax form.

Let's have a look at the important sections of the tax form when it comes to medical expenses.

Line 330 of your income tax form is where you put all the medical expenses you are declaring for yourself, your spouse, your common-law partner, and your dependent children who are under 18 years of age by the end of December 31 of that tax year.

Line 331 of your income tax form is where you put all the medical expenses paid by you or your spouse or common-law partner that you are claiming for other dependants. Dependants in this case are people who depended on you or your spouse or common-law partner for support at some time during the year *and* are one of the following:

- Your children or those of your spouse or your common-law partner, provided they are over 18 (otherwise, their expenses get logged on line 330);
- Your grandchild (or the grandchild of your spouse or your common-law partner);
- Your or your spouse's or common-law partner's parent, grandparent, brother, sister, aunt, uncle, niece, or nephew who was a resident of Canada at any time in the year (friends, no matter how close, don't count).

Tip

When you declare expenses for a dependant (which you declare on line 331) other than your spouse, common-law partner, or minor child (which is line 330), the medical credit calculation is based on their income and not your income. This is very important. If their income is very low, it means that the 3 percent that you need to subtract from the expenses will be very low and you will get approximately a 16 percent tax credit on more of the expense.

Your claim does not need to follow the calendar year like your taxes do. You are allowed to claim expenses over a 12-month period so long as the period ends within the calendar year in which you are filing. For example, if you had an illness starting in the summer of 2005 and you needed a year of rehabilitation that ended in the summer of 2006, you would be allowed to declare all of it on your 2006 tax return—only, of course, if you haven't already declared some of it in 2005.

This is an important point because the more you can declare at once, the more you benefit. Why is this? Because, as discussed above, there is an amount that you have to deduct from your expenses before you can get any credit for them (the 3 percent). So by splitting the expenses into two different years, you are taking that hit twice. It is better to save all your expenses to declare in one year if possible.

Here's an example: Jenny earns $75,000. Three percent of her income is more than $1844, so she would deduct $1844 (since that is the lesser amount) from any medical expense tax credit claim she makes. Jenny has a skiing accident and breaks her leg in several places in April 2005. She needs an operation and extensive physiotherapy. Though the basics are covered by medicare, she decides to use a more aggressive therapy, which she pays for out of her own pocket. Sure enough, by the time she is better, it is August 2006. By now, she has spent $3000 ($2000 in 2005 and another $1000 in 2006). She knows that this is going to be a long process, so she doesn't claim any expenses on her 2005 tax return. This is a wise decision. Below, we will see the two different calculations. The first shows the result if Jenny had claimed her 2005 expenses in 2005 and her 2006 expenses in 2006. The second calculation shows Jenny's claim for the full $3000 in her 2006 income tax return.

Calculation 1: Jenny declares expenses over two years, 2005 and 2006

2005:

Jenny's allowable 2005 expenses	$2000
Deduct	$1844
Difference	$166
Tax credit (approximately 16%)	$26.56

2006:

Jenny's allowable 2006 expenses	$1000

Since $1844 is more than $1000, there is no tax benefit for Jenny at all.

Calculation 2: Jenny declares expenses in 2006

Since Jenny saved her expenses up over a 12-month period that ended in mid-2006, this is what she would declare on her 2006 taxes:

Jenny's allowable expenses over 12 months	$3000
Deduct	$1844
Difference	$1166
Tax credit (16%)	$186

In this case, Jenny would receive a tax credit that is $160 more than in Calculation 1.

Disability Tax Credit

This credit can be claimed by or on behalf of people who qualify as having a severe and prolonged mental or physical impairment, under CRA definitions, which are available on the CRA website. The impairment needs to severely restrict the daily living of the individual, and this condition must be certified by a medical doctor or, if it is sight impairment, an optometrist.

The disability tax credit *cannot* be claimed if you are claiming nursing home care or attendant care toward the calculation of the medical expense tax credit. However, you must qualify for the disability tax credit in order to claim nursing home care or full-time attendant care. Then you have to choose to claim either the disability tax credit or the nursing home care or full attendant care.

To claim the disability tax credit, you must include Form T2201 (Disability Tax Credit Certificate) when filing your income taxes. You can find these on the CRA website under "Forms and Publications" or through your accountant. This form will be reviewed by the CRA to ensure that the person claiming actually qualifies prior to the assessment. If your accountant typically files your return electronically, you will need to inform him or her that you intend to claim this credit. The very first year that you claim it, the tax return will need to be filed the old-fashioned way—by post. After that, electronic filing will be acceptable as long as the impairment is considered permanent.

Here is the calculation:

Amount (fixed by government)	$4233
Times the lowest tax rate (approx.)	16%
Amount of the credit	$720

Note: Rates and amounts may change from year to year.

Who else can claim the disability tax credit? There are others who can claim the disability tax credit for the person with a disability. If you are the supporting person and the person with the disability fits the criteria of a dependant outlined above (see also line 331 of your tax return), then you can claim it. However, there are calculations for how much of this tax credit can be transferred to you, the supporting person. Once again, you need to check with your accountant.

You are also allowed to "divvy up" the disability tax credit between other supporting people. Say you and your brother are the supporting people for your mother. Each of you would be eligible to claim a portion of your mother's disability tax credit (and the other medical expenses associated with her care). But, once again, there are rules. You can never claim more than your mother would have been able to claim herself, and the total claim of you and your brother can't be more than your mother would have claimed. How you divide the claim is up to you and your brother. But no double dipping, which seems to be a common theme in all rules governing income tax deductions and credits!

Tip

Don't assume that if you are entitled to a disability pension under the Canada or Quebec pension plans, you are entitled to this disability tax credit. Different plans have different definitions.

Declaring Expenses for Medical Practitioners

For many of the medical tax credits, certification or prescription by the appropriate medical practitioner is required. In addition, you may claim the services of a medical practitioner. "Medical practitioner" is a term that refers to a broad range of health care providers, including the following:

Doctor
Nurse
Dentist
Pharmacist
Optometrist
Osteopath
Chiropractor
Naturopath
Therapeutist or therapist
Physiotherapist
Chiropodist or podiatrist
Christian Science practitioner
Psychoanalyst
Psychologist
Qualified speech-language pathologist or audiologist
Acupuncturist
Dietitian

Dental hygienist

Occupational therapist

It is important to note that some of the practitioners on this list are not doctors, but their fees can still qualify if they are delivering a "medical service" or a diagnostic, therapeutic, or rehabilitative service.

Tip

Definitions are very important! Remember, the practitioner has to be the *appropriate* practitioner for the treatment, so getting a note from a dental hygienist that certifies your need for an air conditioner won't make the grade.

Also, it is a common mistake to assume that someone is officially certified to perform a function. For example, not every massage therapist is a certified massage therapist. Not everyone who does psychoanalysis is a certified psychoanalyst and therefore eligible to have their services claimed. Always ask and always make sure that their bill includes the certification number or their credentials so that the documentation is valid for the purpose of your tax claim.

Check the list to be sure the practitioner is eligible. The government accepts accreditation by certain colleges and other institutions. A psychologist who received a degree from the Royal College of Silly Walks would not be considered a medical doctor under CRA rules. The CRA list outlines, where applicable, which colleges are accepted.

Plastic surgery performed by a medical doctor, whether in an independent health facility, clinic, or hospital, can be claimed with documented receipts from the medical practitioner.

Medical Expenses Eligible for Tax Credits

The list of what can be claimed as a medical expense is long and subject to redefinition with each federal budget. It is worth checking the CRA's website after each federal budget as well as before filing your annual personal income tax return. If you visit the CRA website, listed in the Resource section, you will be able to access the list of eligible credits. We have highlighted some of what is allowed but the CRA's website is much more detailed. This list is meant to give you a less complicated overview of some of the key claimable medical expenses with some explanatory notes.

Payments to Medical Practitioners and Hospitals

- Claim payments to medical practitioners (see page 203) or to hospitals (public or licensed private hospitals) for medical or dental services provided to you as long as they are not eligible for coverage on your provincial insurance plan or your employer health plan.
- Claim payments made to associations or societies for medical services that they are providing. The example the CRA provides is that of an arthritis sufferer receiving physiotherapy services provided by the Arthritis Society. These are eligible as long as the services are medical and incurred while the patient is at home.

- Out-of-Canada services may be claimable but the CRA will require documentation of the type of institution (the licence it operates with; whether it is officially a hospital, a medical clinic, etc.); the qualifications of the medical professional who saw you; what kind of care you were there for.

Care of an Individual with Mental or Physical Impairment

These expenses can be claimed if the person qualifies for the disability tax credit:

- Claim money paid for one full-time attendant for a patient who has a severe and prolonged mental or physical impairment (see the definitions of these on the CRA website) or for full-time care in a nursing home for such a patient. Note that "full time" doesn't mean one person looking after the patient continuously. It can mean several people covering the care for that person as long as there is only one attendant at any given time. The same is true for the nursing home as long as it provides 24-hour-a-day care by qualified medical personnel. The person providing care for which the claim is being made cannot be under 18 or the spouse or common-law partner of the patient. The patient must qualify for the disability tax credit in order to be able to make this claim.
- A senior who is entitled to the disability credit or who lives in a retirement home can claim up to $10,000

or $20,000 in the year of death. This change was made in 2002.

Note: You cannot claim attendant care as a tax credit if you are claiming it as a deduction (see below).

- Claim amounts up to $10,000 ($20,000 if the person died within the year) for general attendant care of a person qualifying for a disability tax credit. Under this provision, the attendant service doesn't have to be full time. Also, the attendant can be used to provide services that the person with the disability cannot do for him- or herself. Examples are meal preparation, cleaning, transportation services, and even providing companionship to the person with a disability so long as the attendant is doing a little bit of a few things. In short, if the person is employed to do only a specific thing, such as providing maid and cleaning services or transportation services, this would not be viewed by the CRA as attendant care and would not be claimable.
- Claim the amount paid as remuneration for the care and supervision of a person eligible for the disability credit who resides in a home exclusively for such persons.

Tips

When you are paying an attendant directly, he or she must provide you with a receipt that includes his or her social insurance number. These receipts are the supporting documentation that you will need to provide to the CRA.

If you need a full-time attendant, have a doctor write a letter prescribing such care.

Care in an Institution and Training School

- If a doctor certifies that you need specialized training, supervision, or equipment facilities for your condition, these may be claimed. However, the people providing such services in the institution or school need to be specialized to give care to people with your condition. Stop-smoking training is not claimable unless it can be shown that this is part of a bigger health deterioration, and in this case, it must be monitored and prescribed by a medical practitioner.

Transportation and Travel Expenses of Patient and Accompanying Individual

- Ambulances are claimable.
- Other transportation to medical services that are at least 24 miles (40 km) away can be claimed if the route is considered fairly direct, if there is a reasonable need for the service, and if the services are not available closer to the patient.
- You can claim your expenses for your own vehicle or those of a family member if a person who provides professional transportation services is not readily available. This can mean two things. First, there is no readily available commercial vehicle to take you. For example, you call a cab and there is none. Second, the time it will take for the hired vehicle to get you to the medical service is too long and the delay is unaccept-

able. In short, urgency must exist. Claimable expenses are things like mileage.

- Claim the cost of an attendant hired to travel with you if a medical practitioner has certified that you can't travel alone. (Note that some provinces do provide a program for remote areas where some of these costs are covered.)
- Claim other travel expenses, such as meals and accommodation, for both yourself and your attendant for distances over 48 miles (80 km). Once again, it must be shown that there is a need to travel so far and that the route taken was fairly direct.

Expenses to Adapt a Vehicle

- Claim costs to adapt a vehicle used to transport a person who is confined to a wheelchair or the cost for a device that enables a person with a mobility impairment to operate a vehicle (as long as this has been prescribed by a medical practitioner who certifies it as necessary). You can claim up to 20 percent of the cost of an adapted vehicle. Check the CRA website for the rules.

Artificial Limbs, Devices, and Equipment and Products

The list is very extensive, so we are choosing only a few to provide examples:

- Claim the cost of purchased or leased products, equipment, or devices that provide relief, assistance, or treatment for any illness or condition, such as an artificial limb, crutches, an oxygen tent, a guide dog, a van for a wheelchair, or a kidney machine.

- Certain costs associated with these devices, like the special housing for a kidney machine, can be claimed.
- Claim costs related to transportation for the purpose of picking up these devices as long as certain criteria are met and the supplier will not deliver.
- Claim payments for eyeglasses, contact lenses, devices for the treatment or correction of vision, lab tests, and dentures, but only where these have been prescribed by a medical practitioner.
- You can claim 50 percent of the cost of an air conditioner as long as the air conditioner has been prescribed by a medical practitioner for a person with a severe chronic ailment, disease, or disorder. The limit is $1000. For example, a person with multiple sclerosis is very severely affected by heat. A patient could get a physician's note prescribing an air conditioner, which he or she would keep as backup documentation for the claim.
- Claim the cost of products associated with incontinence—diapers, catheter trays and tubes, and disposable briefs are examples of such products.
- Voice-recognition software can be claimed only if the need for such software has been certified in writing by a medical practitioner.

- The cost of guide dogs and hearing dogs and other animals can be claimed. This includes care and maintenance and training for the patient.
- Payments for captioning services or for sign-language interpretation services can be claimed, but only if the payment is provided to a person in the business of providing such a service.
- Claim talking textbooks prescribed by a medical practitioner in connection with an individual's enrolment at an educational institution in Canada, when the individual has a perceptual disability.
- Claim expenses associated with bone marrow or organ transplants, including reasonable legal fees and insurance premiums paid to locate compatible donors or organs, as well as reasonable travel, board, and lodging expenses.
- Claim for drugs and birth control pills prescribed by a doctor and recorded by a pharmacist.
- The cost of dentures can be claimed.
- Claim additional costs related to the purchase of gluten-free food products compared to the cost of comparable non-gluten-free food products for a patient who has celiac disease, provided it has been certified in writing by a medical practitioner.

Premiums

- Claim premiums paid on private health plans other than those paid by your employer.

- Claim deductibles and co-insurance payments (the portion you pay yourself) on provincial drug plans. Any non-reimbursable portion of the cost of insured drugs and services on government and employer plans can be claimed. For example, in Ontario, a seniors' drug plan will cover up to a certain amount of the prescription drug for seniors, and the rest is paid by the senior citizen. The part paid by the senior can be claimed.

Housing and Renovation Costs

- You can claim reasonable expenses incurred for the purpose of moving to a more accessible dwelling, up to a maximum of $2000 by all persons who are making the move.
- Certain renovation costs can be claimed for a person who has a severe and prolonged mobility impairment or who lacks normal physical development. These changes must have been made in order to give that person better access or greater mobility or functioning within the home. This includes additional costs in the actual construction, renovation, or alteration of a principal residence. You cannot claim any rebates you received, including rebates on GST or HST. The CRA gives some good examples of items that can be claimed here, such as the installation of indoor ramps where stairways impede the person's mobility and enlarging doorways or halls to help the person gain access to rooms. (See "What Is

Not Claimable" on page 191 for renovation costs that are not allowed.)

- Claim reasonable moving expenses incurred to move a person with a severe and prolonged condition to housing that is more accessible or allows him or her better mobility or more ability to function.

This list is not meant to be exhaustive, and it is worth navigating the CRA website to double-check on the item you wish to claim and to find out if there are other areas that are less common, and hence not listed here. However, there are a few "must have" principles that you should keep in mind as you review what you can claim and what you can't, and how you go about documenting your need:

1. There must be either a prolonged and severe condition or a clear medical or physical impairment as defined by CRA (for definitions on severe and prolonged impairment, visit the CRA website).
2. There is a clear requirement that the product or service has been certified by a medical doctor or practitioner as defined under the rules of the CRA.
3. No double dipping! You can't claim something that you are eligible to get back somewhere else.
4. Sixteen percent of a reduced amount is not huge. So make sure that these expenses cannot first be submitted to your private health insurance plan, if you have one, or covered by your province or territory in a special program. You can get a much

larger reimbursement than doing it through income tax.

Tip

Always get your medical doctor or practitioner to put in writing what you need and keep this as documentation! It is not enough in an audit to argue that the "doctor told me to buy it."

Attendant Care Deductions

The attendant care deduction is different from the attendant care medical expense tax credit. First, you can deduct from your income payments you make to an attendant. However, you need to qualify for the disability tax credit in order to claim this. The difference is that attendant care expenses, in order to be deducted from your income, need to have been incurred *by you* to enable you to earn income (salary, self-employment, or a training course for which you receive a training allowance). For example, a blind person may employ someone to help him do his job. Perhaps this person would drive him around, escort him places, and help him get information.

Recently, the CRA expanded the attendant care deduction to include certain disability supports such as talking textbooks and sign-language interpreters, but only if they were incurred for education or employment purposes.

Once again, no double dipping. Either you claim these as a deduction *or* you claim these as a medical tax credit—not both.

So what should you do?

Tip

The experts at Grant Thornton suggest in their book *Smart Tax Tips* that if you are disabled and your income is over $35,595, the deduction is worth more to you than the medical tax credit. Take the deduction. A deduction has no threshold, unlike a tax credit, which allows you to claim only the excess over 3 percent of your net income.

Deductions are generally worth more to you than credits. But the attendant care deduction can be claimed only by the person with the disability. In addition, if the person with the disability gets employer-paid allowances or special benefits that enable her to perform her job, these will not be considered personal benefits and added on as income. In short, you will not be taxed on these benefits you receive. For example, people with a sight disability may need transportation to and from work, or if they have problems with mobility, they may need a parking space close to the office. The big test here seems to be reasonableness. The expenses need to be reasonable.

You will need to get form T929—Disability Supports Deduction—fill it out, and submit it with your tax return. (Go to the Forms and Publications section of the CRA website or get the form from your accountant.)

Claiming the Medical Expense Supplemental Refund (Rebate)

A medical expense supplemental refund is actually more like a rebate. So even if you don't owe tax, didn't pay tax, or aren't eligible to get any tax back, you will get this refund back dollar for dollar. Currently, the maximum refund that the government will pay you is $750.

In order to claim this supplement, you must

- be older than 18,
- be a resident of Canada throughout the tax year,
- have claimed medical expenses on line 215 or line 332 of Schedule 1, and
- have an income (employment or net self-employment income must be above $2857).

The calculation for this is a little more tedious. You would calculate 25 percent of all medical expenses that qualify for the medical tax credits, up to a stated maximum. That number is reduced by 5 percent of your family income over $21,663. (Family income means the combined income of you and your spouse or common-law partner.) You will get no more than $750 as refund.

The great news is that you can claim both the medical tax credit *and* the refundable medical expense supplement. Unlike most everything else, it isn't an either/or situation.

There are some circumstances under which you can't claim this supplement. You cannot claim this supplement if your net income (line 236), when combined with the net income of your spouse or common-law partner (line 236 of his or her return, or what it would have been had he or she filed a return), exceeds $36,663.

Tip

If you and your spouse or common-law partner have been separated for more than 90 days, including December of that tax year, his or her income does not have to been included in your calculation. Talk to your accountant about how to ensure that your marital or common-law status is properly reported.

Final Tax Tip

There is a great deal of complexity that has been left out of this chapter that your accountant can help you with. So here's the final tip on this subject: If you would like to claim "grey" areas or other more complicated things, or even if you have questions, do not wait until after January to talk to your accountant. This is the busiest time of year for accountants. They will probably not have the time to sit down with you to sift through all the finer points in the detail required to give you the precise advice you need. And you may not have time to collect all the supporting documentation you need.

What Is Proper Documentation?

You're not going to get very far with the CRA if you don't have proper documentation to support your claims. Medical expenses must be able to be verified by proper receipts. A receipt should include the following information: what the payment was for, the date of the payment, the patient for whom the expense was incurred, and if applicable, the medical practitioner who performed or prescribed the service. For example, if you bought a back brace that was prescribed by your surgeon, the receipt for the brace must indicate that (or the receipt should accompany a letter or note from the surgeon). Cancelled cheques are *not* proper documentation. Accountants will tell you there is a real problem with people assuming that a credit card receipt is adequate documentation. It is not.

Tip

If your doctor says you should get a device, make him or her write out a note on a prescribing pad. That is usually sufficient for a claim.

Vehicle and meal expenses incurred for medical purposes (see below) obviously do not need a doctor's note but the calculation for these expenses must be in accordance with the CRA's method of calculating. Talk to your accountant about this.

Many people file their taxes electronically and submitting these receipts is not possible. It is perfectly acceptable to file your taxes electronically without the receipts, but you must keep them on hand. Often the CRA will ask you to mail in the originals after the fact. So make sure that you have them (and that you copy them before you send them). There is an exception to this. As discussed above, to claim the disability tax credit the first year, you need to provide the appropriate documentation so that the CRA can assess whether you qualify.

Dealing with the Grey Areas

Despite the extensive list of medical expenses eligible for tax credits, situations come up from time to time that aren't neatly defined in the lists provided by the CRA.

Francesca described in Chapter 1 how her daughter had an allergy to milk protein—not a lactose intolerance, which is fairly common, but rather an allergy to milk protein. This condition usually manifests itself close to the start of a baby's life. It is an inability of the lining of the digestive system to handle milk protein. The lining becomes inflamed and the baby passes blood. If untreated, this can result in severe internal bleeding. With time, the system develops and is able to handle milk protein. But while Francesca and her husband waited for their baby's digestive system to "toughen up," they had to put her on a special formula. If the baby is on a regular formula, he or she has to be taken off because it contains milk protein. If the baby is being breastfed, the mother has to avoid anything with milk protein. Francesca was breastfeeding and attempted to alter her eating habits, but she found the diet very restrictive, so she chose to bottle-feed her daughter. The formula was a "denatured" milk product with all the nutrients of regular formulas but no milk protein. The little girl thrived. However, the process to denature milk products is extremely expensive and Francesca was soon spending $80 per week on the formula, or double what regular formula costs. The denatured milk is an over-the-counter product and not covered by any health insurance.

Francesca reviewed the list of eligible medical expenses and noticed that the difference in price between regular and gluten-free products could be claimed by people with celiac disease as a medical tax credit *if* their need has been certified in writing by a medical practitioner. She also noticed that many things on the list required a pharmacist's note or record. Armed with this information, she asked her doctor to write a formal note saying that her child needed this formula for a serious medical condition. She kept this note on file. She also asked him to provide a prescription for the formula and she also kept that on file.

Each time she bought the formula, she would ask the pharmacist for a handwritten prescription receipt. (Because the product is not a prescription drug, it therefore is not entered in the prescription computer system, so no computerized receipt could be printed.) She kept all the receipts and at the end of the year claimed the difference between the special formula and regular formula.

The formula met another criterion set out by the CRA: Products are eligible if a person without such impairment would not incur the cost to buy them. Although Francesca was enthusiastic about the particular product, she does not believe it is a formula that any parent would use if he or she didn't absolutely have to for medical reasons. It didn't dissolve as easily as the regular formula did. It didn't smell or taste as good as the regular formula. It wasn't any more nutritious than regular formula, and it cost twice as much.

Such claims are in the "grey" area. If you wish to claim, keep all the documentation, however, in case it ever does become an issue.

Another example can be drawn from a friend's pregnancy. She enlisted a doula to help her. (See Chapter 1, "Having a Baby in Canada.") Doulas are not on the list of claimable medical practitioners. However, her doula was also a registered nurse. *Could she claim or not?*

Our friend Joanne claimed the expense based on this reasoning: "I didn't hire her to help me set up the nursery or pick names for the baby. I hired her to help me deliver my baby, to help me recognize the signs of potential problems. In fact, her nursing expertise was probably more crucial to me than her doula training." The mother claimed her as a nursing aide. The doula put all her credentials on her bill. Our friend realizes now, though, that her benefit plan would have covered the doula's services because she is a registered nurse and she has a registered nurse's number. Claiming the nurse/doula on her benefit plan would have been far more beneficial to Joanne than declaring her services as a medical expense. Joanne would have been reimbursed for most of her fee rather than receiving only a marginal percentage of a percentage as a credit against taxes. Always check whether the service or product is claimable on your benefit plan first.

Tips

Where there are grey areas and you feel very strongly about an expense, there is nothing stopping you from claiming it on your tax return. However, here are the things you need to do:

1. Be reasonable—don't stretch too far.
2. For services you need, enlist, where possible, a health care practitioner who is among the certified practitioners on the list. If the service itself isn't specifically listed, you can be certain it will be a hard sell.
3. Double-check with your accountant when in doubt and be certain to mention the credentials of the practitioners.
4. Document! Almost all items you can claim need a doctor's note or prescription. Make certain your medical practitioner has provided you with something saying that this item is necessary for your medical condition.
5. Be prepared to defend your claim with a solid argument.
6. Full details on medical expense and disability tax credits and attendant care expense deductions can be found on the CRA website. This document is rather complicated and provides the interpretation of these claims. Your accountant may understand some of the areas better than you will. Still, it is good to know where these things are found. Where there is a grey area, it is not a bad idea to print out the portion of the interpretation you think might be relevant. The accountant can help you make a determination.

Despite the CRA's excellent and extensive lists, they are not exhaustive. There are still many judgment calls that need to be made, as evidenced by the many court cases dealing with areas that are not entirely clear. Health care professionals are not always the best people to ask for advice on whether you can claim their services. They may not be up to date with the latest amendments and expansions of the medical expense tax credit list.

No one can predict what an audit will conclude, but the CRA is generally reasonable. However, should they in their wisdom disagree with your viewpoint, you will be required to pay the tax that you would have paid had you not claimed.

Just to summarize the sometimes complex information given in this chapter, here are the basics to help you. There is much that you can declare as medical expenses, provided you keep the proper documentation. There is more that can be declared as credits or deductions if you or your dependant qualifies as a person with a disability or severe and prolonged impairment.

Things to do:

1. Review the CRA definitions to see if you or a family member qualifies as a person with a disability or severe or prolonged impairment.
2. Make sure that you obtain from the CRA the forms you will need.
3. Ask for receipts for everything and review them immediately to ensure they contain the information the CRA requires.

In addition:

1. Leave no stone unturned and think, think, think! If you are a disabled person, does your employer

provide you with a benefit that enables you to do your job? If so, make sure your accountant knows so that you are not paying taxable benefits!

2. Be reasonable, and be prepared!
3. Try to claim on your benefit plan first! It is far more beneficial to you.

RESOURCE GUIDE

BOOKS

Smart Tax Tips. Grant Thornton and Karen Yull (Toronto: Key Porter, 2005).

This is simply the best book we have found that deals with all kinds of tax areas. It provides tips on income taxes and has an excellent section dedicated to medical expenses. It is frequently updated to reflect the latest government budget changes as they affect the tax rules. You can order this from your Grant Thornton representative office or get it at your local bookstore. Grant Thornton's website will give you a complete listing of its offices in Canada: www.grantthornton.ca.

ORGANIZATIONS AND GOVERNMENT PROGRAMS

The Canadian Diabetes Association
www.diabetes.ca
Telephone: 1-800-BANTING (226-8464)
In the section of the website called "News Releases," this

association provides excellent information on making claims for people with diabetes.

Canada Revenue Agency
www.cra-arc.gc.ca
Telephone for income tax inquiries: 1-800-959-8281
TTY: 1-800-665-0354
This agency used to be called Revenue Canada. It is the definitive source of information with regard to what you can and cannot declare, although the website has been a little out of date on recent changes in the federal budget. Still, it is a very important source for information on taxes. Your accountant will be sent all the recent updates.

Navigating the CRA Website

Click on "About Your Tax Return." Then click on "Completing." Click on "What You Can Deduct." In the next window, select "M" for medical expenses. Scroll down and you will see a list of all the areas regarding medical expenses. Choose the area you would like to know more about.

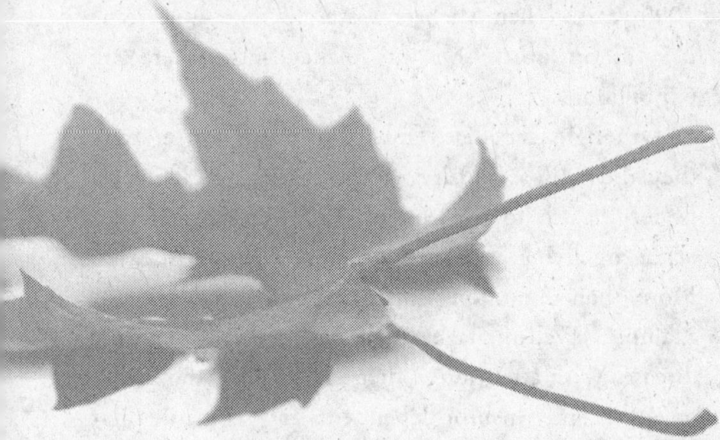

Managing Aging

We Canadians have the problem in health care that we have always wanted. What do we mean by that? Well, we wanted to live longer, and life expectancy in Canada has grown dramatically. In the 1920s, Canadians lived into their mid-50s. By the 1950s, Canadians were living into their mid-60s. And now Canadian life expectancy has expanded further. Most Canadians will live into their late 70s or their 80s or even their 90s. According to Statistics Canada, more than 4700 Canadians now living have already reached the age of 100. So we have the outcome we wanted—a longer life—except now we have the problem that goes with it: managing chronic disease. On a worldwide basis, life expectancy has expanded more in the past 40 years than in the previous

2000 years. When Michael was born, there were some 2.5 billion others on our planet—now there are 6.5 billion.

Although Canadians are living much longer than they did half a century ago, they are not living in perfect health to the end of their life. Rather, they often are living with one or more chronic diseases. More than 2 million Canadians have diabetes, for example. Well-managed diabetes is truly a chronic disease. With attention to diet and exercise, those who have become insulin-dependent can control their blood sugar levels through tough-minded and careful management. Professional athletes, such as hockey player Bobby Clarke, who have led active lives while managing their diabetes are proof it can be done. Sadly, there are also tens of thousands of Canadians for whom poorly managed diabetes has resulted in unnecessary amputation of limbs, heart disease, blindness, and other consequences.

Much the same is true of other chronic diseases, including asthma, arthritis, and chronic heart disease. Appropriate diet and exercise, coupled with medical intervention, such as the right drugs at the right time, can make your longer life a happy and healthy one. Your ability to navigate your chronic disease depends on these same principles. It's important to have as much information about your disease as possible. We will focus on managing chronic disease in Chapter 8 and coping with cancer in Chapter 9. Prior to managing chronic disease or cancer, many Canadians of the baby-boom generation will face other health challenges. How to maintain a boomer body? How to prepare for the long haul? These topics are tackled in Chapter 7, "Boomer Maintenance."

SEVEN

Boomer Maintenance

The baby-boom generation—those people born between the late 40s and early 60s—is starting to hit the health system. Fortunately, most boomers are not hitting the health system with life-threatening heart disease, cancer, or strokes—at least, not yet! Baby boomers are turning up in the health care system in increasing numbers because of bad maintenance on the boomer body. Lower back pain, diminished vision, hearing loss, sore knees, and overwhelmingly those extra pounds that have been packed on are all real issues for boomers. Navigating the health system for boomers is about maintenance and avoidance, two closely related ideas. Maintenance is about taking care of yourself so you can avoid chronic disease or really serious illnesses later on. In fact, your approach to maintaining yourself physically in the boomer years will have a lot to do with the quality of life you enjoy in your 60s, 70s, 80s, and 90s. You need to take good care of all your moving parts:

your heart, your lungs, your back, your joints, and your eyes. As those of us who are baby boomers move into our middle years, we begin to be aware that our bodies aren't functioning quite as well as they used to. Let's look at some of the areas that commonly are of concern at this stage of life.

Tip

Get yourself a comprehensive guide to your health. Use small illnesses and injuries as an excuse to read and learn about your health. Two excellent guides, one from Harvard Medical School and one from the University of Toronto Faculty of Medicine, are listed at the end of this chapter.

The Annual Checkup versus the Periodic Health Exam

Michael was surprised to learn during his service as Ontario's Deputy Minister of Health that the annual medical was not universally recommended. Even though it was an insured service and doctors were paid to perform annual medicals, the scientific community favoured the periodic health examination. He asked what the difference was. The answer was that not everyone needs the same tests annually. Depending on family and personal medical history, as well as age, gender, and physical condition, you might need a variety of tests every year but certain others only every two, three, or five years. In the 1990s Canada even had a Task

> **Tip**
>
> Get a personalized periodic health examination. Discuss with your doctor your personal risk factors based on your own family history and lifestyle. Get advice on how to lower your risk factors.

Force on Periodic Health Examinations. Later that task force became the Canadian Task Force on Preventative Health Care, a broader concept. Still later, its funding was cut and its very useful work ended. What does this mean for you?

Certainly regular testing for a variety of conditions is warranted. How frequently and for what varies. For example, if your mother and grandmother had breast cancer, your mammogram should be more frequent. If your father or mother had colorectal cancer, you should be tested at a younger age and perhaps more frequently than is normal. If there is a family history of diabetes, your weight and blood sugar levels are early indicators of your risk—they need to be tested. Elevated blood pressure is a warning sign for both heart disease and stroke.

Your Heart

The number-one cause of illness, disability, and death in Canada remains diseases of the heart and circulatory system. The good news is that progress has been made. Hospital admissions related to heart disease dropped from 1695 per 100,000 population in 1994–95 to 1339 in 2001–02 for those over 20 years of age. The trend continued with admissions for new heart attacks dropping by 19 percent from 1999 to 2005. Strokes were down 23 percent in the same period. We are living longer with healthier hearts but—and this is the bad news—heart disease is still risk factor number one. What can you do to lessen your chances of heart and circulatory problems?

The Heart and Stroke Foundation Canada has identified seven risk factors associated with heart disease.

Risk Factors

You can't control who your parents are and what genes they gave you. But luckily, you can control several factors that could increase your risk of heart disease and stroke, such as obesity, diet, diabetes, smoking, high blood pressure, and high cholesterol.

1. OBESITY

People who are overweight or obese risk developing high blood pressure, high blood lipids, and diabetes—all of which put them at high risk of cardiovascular or heart disease. If you are concerned about your weight or your doctor has expressed concern, talk to him or her about a diet that will bring your weight under control. Ask about exercise and what level of physical activity you should be attempting. Remember, you're trying to stay out of the health care system for as long as possible—just one visit with your family doctor can provide you with valuable information that could forestall frequent and lengthy interactions with the health care system in the future. Extreme measures for losing weight include various kinds of surgery, such as what is called "stomach stapling," but it is far, far better to start with diet and exercise to control your weight.

2. CHOLESTEROL

Cholesterol is a soft waxy substance manufactured by human and animal bodies. There are different types of cholesterol and different particle sizes. The details of the science are best left to researchers, but what you need to know is that "bad" cholesterol—also known as low density lipoprotein (LDL)—clogs your arteries, increasing your risk of heart disease and stroke. The "good" cholesterol, or high-density lipoprotein particles (HDL), actually helps clean excess cholesterol out of your bloodstream. You should be tested for cholesterol as part of your periodic health examination. Get a good explanation of how changes in your diet and more exercise can reduce the bad cholesterol in your body. These changes take time, so avoid frequent testing as it will not show very much change.

Tip

Ask your doctor to explain your cholesterol test results and what you can do to lower bad cholesterol. A nurse or dietitian can also give good advice.

3. DIABETES

Diabetes occurs when your body can't process sugar properly. Juvenile diabetes, or type 1 diabetes, which develops in childhood and continues for the individual's lifetime, is treated with insulin. Adult onset diabetes, or type 2 diabetes, often develops in people who are overweight. There is no such thing as having a bit of diabetes—you either have it or you don't. At your periodic health examination your doctor will test your blood for indicators of diabetes. The long-term consequences of diabetes, particularly badly managed diabetes, are not pleasant. Diabetics suffer increased heart disease. The most severe consequences are the amputation of limbs and blindness. The risk of adult onset diabetes can be reduced by exercise, diet, and maintaining a reasonable body weight.

4. SMOKING

Smoking is a dangerous health hazard that is the single most important cause of preventable illness and premature death for Canadians. Smoking is not only damaging to the heart but also the primary cause of lung cancer.

Tip

Your doctor can help you stop smoking by recommending stop smoking programs or suggesting medication that will help.

5. PHYSICAL ACTIVITY

A sedentary lifestyle (read: couch potato behaviour) can lead directly to heart and circulatory problems. Regular aerobic physical activity is a great asset to keeping your heart healthy and leading a healthy lifestyle. Before you start on any increased physical activity, visit your doctor for a full assessment and advice about the level of activity you are capable of. It doesn't take long to see the benefits of increased physical activity.

> **Tip**
>
> Remember the pedometer we talked about earlier? Walking is one of the easiest and most satisfying ways of getting exercise—and getting fit.

6. SMOG

New research shows that air pollution is a serious heart disease risk. During the hot, hazy days of summer—otherwise known as primetime smog season—learn from reading and from your doctor or nurse how you can protect your heart health. You can't always change where you live and you certainly can't change the weather, but taking a few precautions will lessen the stress on your heart.

Tip

If you have asthma or other respiratory problems, avoid the outdoors on high smog-alert days.

7. HIGH BLOOD PRESSURE

One of the key risk factors for heart disease and stroke is high blood pressure. Your doctor will check your blood pressure. You can also test your own blood pressure at many pharmacies or, with the proper equipment, at home.

Tip

Your doctor is your best adviser on what mix of exercise, diet, and medications will reduce your blood pressure. Make medications your last resort, not your first resort, as diet changes and exercise will have other benefits.

Preventing Diabetes

What are the consequences for you if you are living with diabetes? What are the consequences if you are diagnosed with diabetes in the future? First, there is the disease itself and its impacts. But the complications that can result from the disease are even more serious. It may surprise you to learn that in Ontario, people with diabetes make up only 7.5 percent of the population but account for 32 percent of heart attacks, 30 percent of strokes, 51 percent of new dialysis cases, and 70 percent of limb amputations.

As we mentioned, there are two types of diabetes. Type 1 is the inherited type and counts for only 10 percent of diabetics. The dramatic growth is for people with type 2 diabetes. Here is the good news: You can prevent or delay type 2 diabetes through increased physical activity, healthy eating, weight loss, not smoking, and stress reduction. One study showed that people at risk for type 2 diabetes were able to cut that risk by 58 percent by doing two things: exercising moderately for 30 minutes a day and losing 5 to 7 percent of their body weight. For people over 60, the effects were even greater—their risk was cut by almost 71 percent. These results have been found in other similar studies.

Tip

Understand your risks for developing diabetes and take concrete steps to lower them. This is a disease you really, really want to avoid if possible.

Your Lower Back

Many people in their middle years experience lower back pain. The first stop in the search for relief is usually the family doctor for a prescription. For most people, drugs are the first solution to lower back pain. Other remedies are heating pads, cooling pads, and all manner of similar interventions. The advice offered here is somewhat different. The first stop you should make is the nearest bookstore to buy a copy of Dr. Hamilton Hall's spectacular book *The Back Doctor*. Dr. Hall is one of Canada's leading spine surgeons, a co-founder of the Canadian Back Institute and a chain of clinics specializing in backs, and a thoughtful author. Even if you consult with your doctor about your back problems, you should be fully informed on all aspects of back care. Dr. Hall estimates that 80 to 90 percent of back surgeries are unnecessary as there are other ways of getting the same result.

The causes of back pain are varied and sometimes mysterious, as Michael learned early in his life. When he was young, his surgeon father would take him along on Saturday morning hospital rounds at the four or five hospitals where he had privileges. One Saturday they were confronted by a patient in clear agony. He demanded, "Doc, when can I have my surgery?" Michael's father's reply was terse: "We will see."

As they drove to the next hospital, Michael's father commented that his patient owned a car dealership. At the next hospital they found another middle-aged man, also in agony with a sore back. He too wanted to know when Michael's father could perform his surgery. He got the same terse answer: "We will see."

To Michael's astonishment his father told him the second patient was also a car dealership owner. There seemed to be an epidemic of back pain among car dealership owners!

Finally, his father explained. "Every year these two dealers have to put in their order for new cars. The stress is intense. They develop extreme back pain. If they order too many cars, they can go broke. If they order too few, they miss sales."

"When will you do their surgery?" Michael asked.

"Never!" was his surgeon father's answer. "After they decide on their order, their backs get better and they go home."

It was an important early lesson in the relationship between stress and the human body.

Tip

Eight out of 10 people will have significant back pain sometime in their life. Some will choose to suffer and others will opt for surgery that may not be necessary. Know your options and what you can expect from the treatment you choose.

Another story about backs illustrates how surgery can be avoided. Michael's father had a cottage next door to a lawyer who was a little on the heavy side. This fellow appeared at Michael's father's office one day, clutching his back, and began to take off his shirt so he could be examined. "Keep your shirt on, Sidney" was the response. The lawyer was startled. Michael's father said, "I sit on the end of my dock and watch you run up those 200 steps from the lake to your cottage every weekend. Sell the cottage, Sidney. That will fix your back."

All sorts of things cause pain in the lower back and all sorts of things remedy it. In fact, a major study undertaken in the United States by the Agency for Healthcare Research and Quality, a national research agency, indicated that a range of interventions—medications, physical therapy, massage therapy, chiropractic treatment, back surgery, even doing nothing—had all produced roughly the same results. The powers that be in the medical profession and the pharmaceutical industry were so incensed by this study that they came close to having the agency closed down. And yet there is huge truth in the finding. Every case is different, of course, and if you're having back trouble, you shouldn't ignore it. But before you embark on painful surgery or expensive physiotherapy, read through Dr. Hall's book so you're as informed as you can be about back problems. And if any of the therapies make you feel better, there's nothing wrong with that!

These are the years when you can't be quite as cavalier as you used to be where your back is concerned—you'd best take care of it. You should also think through which of the available interventions is the one that's going to serve you the best in the decades ahead. Surgery is a one-time deal. The advantage of surgery is that it may relieve a patient's constant and intense pain. However, this result is not always achieved. A disadvantage may be a loss of flexibility, resulting in a permanently stiff back. If you can manage to improve your back and eliminate pain in other ways, you will have maintained the flexibility that evolution intended for your back. We are not suggesting that all back surgery should be avoided—there are many important instances where it is absolutely the right thing to do.

Tip

Know your back—take care of your back and watch your back!

Your Hips and Knees

Even before your hips and knees start to give you trouble, you'll be well aware they could cause trouble on two fronts: the physical discomfort and outright pain, and the challenge of getting treatment. In discussions about the health care system, much of the talk and writing has centred on wait times for hip and knee replacements. Here's a simple piece of advice for boomers: Rather than wait impatiently on a list for new knees and hips, take some weight off and keep the originals. The major cause of the degeneration of hip and knee joints is arthritis. That disease can be made worse by inactivity and by obesity.

Managing arthritis is the best means of preventing or deferring your need for joint replacement. The Arthritis Society (www.arthritis.ca) offers the sensible advice of moderation: moderation in exercise for those living with arthritis, and moderation in your weight. You'll find more on arthritis in Chapter 8, "Tips for Managing Chronic Disease."

Here are a few facts about weight and hip and knee problems:

- Obese Canadians are three times more likely to have a hip or knee replacement than people who are not overweight.
- Nearly 9 of 10 knee-replacement patients were overweight or obese.
- Seven of 10 hip-replacement patients were overweight or obese.

Tip

Consider the wear and tear from carrying the extra pounds and take steps to lose them. If you need to have replacement surgery, look for a centre of excellence that does lots of hip and knee replacements. Be willing to wait a little to get an excellent outcome. Try to lose excess pounds while you are waiting.

Your Eyes

When Michael was a child, his surgeon father forced him and his five brothers and sisters to eat carrots. "They will improve your night vision," he declared. As an adult, Michael learned that during World War II, the British, in an effort to hide the newly invented radar from the Germans, put about word that the accuracy of their night raids was due to carrot consumption by pilots. Many years later Michael discovered that science had caught up with his father's advocacy—carrots, spinach, melons, and citrus are all proclaimed by Health Canada to slow age-related eye diseases such as cataracts, macular degeneration, and glaucoma.

In addition to eating carrots, you can take several other steps to protect your vision:

- You can stop smoking. Apparently the smoke does get in your eyes and can trigger the early onset of age-related macular degeneration, a disease that causes permanent loss of central vision.
- When you are outdoors, get yourself sunglasses that block both UV-A and UV-B rays that can damage your eyes. Wear them.
- As our parents always advocated, read in good light.
- Be careful when undertaking any activity that involves cutting or other activities that can cause eye injury.
- After age 45, get a regular eye examination as part of your periodic health exam.

Cataracts

Cataracts are a natural part of aging. In this disease the lens of the eye gradually becomes cloudy and your vision also becomes cloudy. Fortunately, there is a surgical procedure to remove cataracts. It is the most frequently performed surgery—over 250,000 cataract surgeries are performed annually in Canada, all of them covered by medicare. Governments across the country allocate more funds for cataract surgeries than for any other surgery.

RESOURCE GUIDE

BOOKS

Either of these two comprehensive health guides should be a part of your ongoing education about your body and the various ailments you and your family will face:

The Complete Canadian Health Guide: Revised and Updated. June Engel, ed. (Toronto: Key Porter, 2005).

Endorsed by the University of Toronto's Faculty of Medicine, Canada's largest medical faculty, this guide brings together the expertise of hundreds of medical experts in a single 608-page volume.

Harvard Medical School Family Health Guide. Anthony L. Komaroff, ed. (New York: Simon & Shuster, 2004).

A Consultation with the Back Doctor. Hamilton Hall (Toronto: McClelland & Stewart, 2003).

Dr. Hall advocates for activity rather than bed rest, independent knowledge rather than dependence on a health professional, and a common sense approach. This is essential reading for anyone who has back pain or wishes to avoid back pain. You get only one spine—this is the owner's manual.

Consumer Health Information Service—Toronto Reference Library
www.tpl.toronto.on.ca/uni_chi_index.jsp
Telephone: (416) 393-7056 or 1-800-667-1999
789 Yonge Street, 3rd Floor
Toronto, Ontario
M4W 2G8
This service is to the best of our knowledge unique. It is dedicated to giving people access to health information. Even if you don't live in Toronto, you can visit the website and take advantage of the on-line information it provides. It includes links to expert sites. However, there are public libraries in every city and town across Canada. All of them stock books on health and wellness. Your librarian is an excellent guide to finding the information you need. You can also use a service called inter-library loan, which allows books to travel among libraries to meet your needs.

At the time of writing, the Toronto Reference Library was updating its "Health Navigators," which are brief guides to sources of information on a variety of health topics. They serve as a useful starting point when you're looking for health information. Check in at www.tpl.toronto.on.ca/ uni_chi_finder.jsp to find out if the Health Navigators have a new home.

ORGANIZATIONS AND ASSOCIATIONS

Heart and Stroke Foundation of Canada
www.heartandstroke.ca
This terrific website offers lots of advice, from ideas for healthy eating to interactive tools to manage your stress, stop smoking, and maintain a healthy weight.

Canadian Diabetes Association
www.diabetes.ca
The website presents very solid information on diabetes and on all aspects of living with diabetes, from dental care to exercise to travel tips and complications.

College of Family Physicians
www.cfpc.ca
The College offers an excellent Patient Education Program. Its website has fact sheets on 68 separate topics of interest to patients and to those trying to stay healthy.

Among the issues covered are these:

Acne in Teens: Ways to control it
Breast Cancer: Steps to find breast lumps early
Cholesterol: What you can do to lower your level
Diabetes: Taking charge of your diabetes
Low Back Pain: Tips on pain relief and prevention
Weight Control: Losing weight and keeping it off

The Eyecare Trust
www.eye-care.org.uk
The Eyecare Trust was originally known as the Eyecare Information Service. It was set up to act as an independent source of information on all eye-related issues and to raise public awareness about the importance of regular eye care.

GOVERNMENT PROGRAMS

Public Health Agency of Canada
www.phac-aspc.gc.ca
The relatively new Public Health Agency of Canada was born out of the SARS epidemic, but it has a great deal of very useful advice on health issues beyond infectious diseases. Of particular interest are the publications and guides available on the site. For example, there is a free physical activity guide with a range of tips for increasing your level of physical activity. There are also over 100 publications. Some are obscure and for experts, but many are for Canadians looking for information on how to stay healthy. Info sheets on everything from foot care to vision care are provided as well as advice in a readable series, It's Your Disease, that covers a wide range of topics.

EIGHT

Tips for Managing Chronic Disease

The reality of our time is that we are living much longer than previous generations. However, we are living longer not in perfect health but with an array of chronic diseases, such as diabetes, asthma, heart disease, and arthritis. As we saw in the previous chapter, hundreds of thousands of Canadians will experience vision loss owing to treatable conditions, and still others will require joint replacements to their hips and their knees to be able to walk without excruciating pain. Mental illness and related addictions will afflict millions of Canadians, resulting in both incapacity and societal stigma. Managing these diseases and conditions well is the major challenge facing the Canadian health system. Managing these diseases will also be your biggest challenge as you age.

This chapter provides some tips for managing your chronic diseases and navigating the emerging network of information and organized supports. Some of the major chronic diseases are tackled in more detail. You should be aware that the advice offered herein is not medical advice. Rather, it is advice about the benefits of better knowledge and better management. It is also a guide to resources that can assist you in navigating the chronic diseases that may be your intimate companions through life's journey.

If we try to manage chronic disease in the existing hospital system, the most likely outcomes will be excessive costs and poor results. The struggle is to find better ways of managing these diseases in the home and the community. Fortunately there is an abundance of evidence that better management equals better outcomes for you.

Chronic Disease—By the Numbers

Managing chronic disease is a growing challenge as we age. Statistics Canada provides the following overview (see p. 252) based on its National Population Health Survey. It shows the percentage of the Canadian population who is reporting various chronic disease at age 65 and also between ages 45 and 64. The overall picture is one of a mounting burden as the population ages.

As you can see, aging produces significant increases in rates of heart disease, hypertension, activity limitation, and diabetes. The only modest decrease is in migraine headaches. But the trend is clear. We are an aging population with a mounting burden of chronic disease.

Chronic Condition/ Disease	Canadians Affected 1998/99 (%)	
	Age 45–64	Age 65+
Arthritis/Rheumatism	19.9%	41.5%
Hypertension	16.2%	35.6%
Heart Disease	4.8%	17.4%
Diabetes	5.1%	11.6%
Bronchitis	2.1%	5.8%
Asthma	5.8%	5.7%
Migraine Headaches	7.5%	3.3%
Activity Limitations	16.2%	29.1%

The World Health Organization provides a sobering global perspective: "The world is experiencing a rapid rise in chronic health problems to the extent that chronic conditions now account for over half of the global disease burden. Previously, acute infectious diseases were the primary focus of the healthcare workforce in every country. However, during the past century, advances in medical science, technology and public health, such as immigrations, sanitation, housing and education, have contributed to a decrease in acute diseases. As a result, life expectancy has risen during this period."

If we consider the close linkage of hypertension and heart disease, as well as the reality that bronchitis and asthma are both respiratory ailments, then our list consolidates into four major chronic disease clusters:

- Diabetes
- Arthritis
- Respiratory (asthma/bronchitis)
- Heart disease/hypertension

After some general tips on navigating chronic disease, we turn our attention in this chapter to the four major chronic diseases. We also talk about mental illnesses, which can be chronic and debilitating. Don't be despondent if your disease is not among the top four—the same general advice has merit. Find knowledgeable professionals, become educated about your chronic disease, find the website of the related association, and seek out an organized program of care and self-management.

At a conference on the management of chronic disease, held in Toronto in 2006, experts agreed that prevention and healthy living are essential in order to avoid chronic disease in the first place. Many millions of Canadians, though, will spend decades dealing with one or more chronic diseases because of our very human failings and our straying from a healthy life. Chronic disease also rests on the foundation of our genetic code—what has come down to us through evolution and our family tree.

Tip

Stay healthy through active living and a healthy diet. This will better equip you to cope with whatever chronic conditions afflict you.

Are We Receiving the Best Care for Chronic Disease?

The simple answer is that not all of us are. A recent study by the Commonwealth Fund, a private foundation whose aim is to improve health care systems, compared two chronic diseases and their treatment across six nations.

Adults Who Had Proper Testing in the Last Year

	% for Hypertension	% for Diabetes
Canada	85	38
Australia	78	41%
New Zealand	77	40
U.K.	72	58
U.S.	85	56
Germany	91	55

As you can see, 85 percent of Canadians with hypertension received the standard of care recommended by experts. Fifteen percent, or 1 in 6, did not.

In the case of diabetes, the findings are far worse. Only 38 percent of Canadian diabetic patients are receiving the recommended annual care, which includes eye and foot examinations as well as hemoglobin and cholesterol testing. So 62 percent, or more than 6 in 10, did not have the required testing.

Canada does not perform dramatically better or worse than other industrialized nations. But for you, the patient, this should be an important wake-up call. This is why you need to take responsibility for managing your chronic disease.

Dr. Paul Wallace of Kaiser Permanente, a large and well-regarded American health maintenance organization, put it this way: You may spend 15 minutes four times a year with your doctor, or a total of one hour. The other 8759 hours a year you will be managing your disease! Self-management is at the core of the new and more successful approaches.

Tip

Take control and educate yourself to self-manage! Get training in self-management for your disease. You can locate it through your local health authority or the website of the disease-specific group.

Dr. Wallace went on to note that patients are not eager to be coached by their doctor about how to cope with their illness. We are much more comfortable being coached by a nurse or a pharmacist. Apparently, we are uncomfortable taking up the time of a busy physician.

It has been found that very specific and organized disease-management programs get better results than any other approach. This type of "tight" management requires frequent testing to ensure proper treatment. It means taking the required medication at exactly the right time. It also means fully utilizing the positive impacts of proper diet and exercise to improve your condition. Tight management also means having a team of providers to back you up. The alternative to tight management and an organized program of disease management with a multi-disciplinary team is all too often the harried family doctor. Some family doctors do a superb job of managing diabetes or asthma. Most family doctors are generalists and will refer you to a specialist. The notion of the team is that it gives the family doctor more ability to orchestrate your care without being the sole provider of it.

How much better are the outcomes from tight management? Dr. David Crookston, a family doctor with the Group Health Centre (GHC) in Sault Ste. Marie, Ontario, long a model of organized care, reported results from a program to treat congestive heart failure. By organizing more comprehensive care, including a multi-disciplinary team and an electronic health record, the GHC reduced heart patients' hospital readmissions within one month of heart attacks from over 40 percent to under 5 percent. Hospital readmission rates are a valuable measure of the quality of care the patient receives. If the readmission rate is high (such as 40 percent) it suggests that the care is episodic and on a crisis basis. A low readmission rate (such as 5 percent) suggests that the disease is being well managed in the home and community setting. Outcomes also improved dramatically for the over 3000 patients managing diabetes with the support of a team approach at GHC.

Tip

Seek out an organized program for chronic disease management. Enrol in it if you can. Look for programs by contacting your disease-specific association, by asking your family doctor, and by reviewing websites such as that of your provincial department of health.

All across Canada innovative leaders in health care are successfully taking up the challenge of chronic disease. Dr. Art McGregor, a leading family physician and innovator from Victoria, described his team approach for managing chronic disease. The group began with 30 family physicians and two nurses and has expanded to 65 family doctors in 33 different offices. At the core of its success are monitoring, assessments, and measurement of specific indicators, including hard results from the lab and softer indications from clinical examinations. For the patient this means more intensive testing, monitoring, and a larger self-management role. The benefit is a healthier patient and fewer complications from the chronic disease.

At present this is not the approach offered in all or even most primary care settings. You will need to ask your doctor and look around your community to find this type of care. It is well worth the search. For diabetes, testing rates improved to nearly double the average in British Columbia. Outcomes for patients showed significant improvement.

If you are a diabetic or an asthmatic or someone who has a family history of any chronic disease, you should be a strong supporter of these reforms. Only with a more robust and organized approach on the part of the health care community will all the benefits of modern health care be felt by those living with chronic disease.

You need to learn as much as you can about the disease or diseases that you will be managing for the rest of your life. You will be the key manager, but with the changes to the medical system, you can build a team to coach and support you. As you start to take responsibility for the management of your condition, look for innovative approaches and family health teams that can support you. One thing to look for is a clinic or primary care group that uses an electronic health record system.

We talked about the advantages of electronic health records in Chapter 4. They save health care professionals money and time. But why should you care as a patient?

There are some clear advantages for patients. A Danish study of the move from paper records to electronic prescribing found that there were fewer problems with prescriptions. In the paper world, 33 percent, or one in three prescriptions, caused a problem of one sort or another. With electronic prescribing, where the prescription moves electronically from doctor to pharmacy, the problem rate dropped to 14 percent, or less than one in seven. Not perfect, but way better for you as a patient. Rates of electronic prescribing are increasing in Canada but still represent the minority of prescriptions written.

Tip

Electronic records do not guarantee safer, higher-quality care, but they do help avoid errors. Look for a health provider organization—a primary care team or a family doctor—that has an electronic health record system.

Dr. David Bates is chief of general medicine at the prestigious Brigham and Women's Hospital, affiliated with the Harvard Medical School in Boston, Massachusetts. In a presentation to a conference on the electronic health record, he supported the benefits to the patient. Dr. Bates noted that when paper records were used, the average patient encounter lasted 12 minutes and the average time to the first interruption by the physician was 18 seconds. In these encounters patients reported that 75 percent of the time they left with unanswered questions. Dr. Bates noted that an electronic record with prompts and alerts to specific issues allows far more to be accomplished in a physician–patient encounter. The old paper record is being replaced with a much more modern electronic record. Doctors, nurses, and other health professionals can enter data in a variety of ways. A desktop computer is one method, and so are such devices as Palm Pilots and BlackBerrys. As well, doctors can access patient records from their home and receive test results electronically. X-rays and MRIs now move as electronic files rather than the old days of film. This enables faster transmission from radiologist to attending physician.

In Britain, the National Health Service is moving from a physician booking hospital appointments for patients to patients themselves booking appointments. The doctor determines that the patient needs, for example, an ultrasound. Rather than engaging in a flurry of phone calls, the patient is able to access the schedule of available appointments over the Internet and select a convenient appointment time. This parallels the Internet booking of air travel that most major airlines have adopted. Using a computer, patients go to a main website and select which hospital they wish to go to, or they do the same thing through a phone call to a special appointments line.

Canada is moving toward these systems in fits and starts, and you should monitor whether they have reached your province or community. In pockets across the country, you can find innovative methods of handling your medical file that involve you. The day is not far off when we will have the same ability as Danish patients to access our own medical records. In 2005, Danish patients were able to view their own records and even contribute their own information, such as their height and weight. In the meantime, though, most of us are still dealing with medical professionals who work with paper.

Whether your doctor uses paper or electronic systems to track your records, the following five tips are common to managing chronic diseases. Keep them in mind as you review the specific information for your chronic disease.

1. Know your disease—know as much about the disease as possible. Develop good information sources, both on the Internet and from some of the resource books listed at the end of this chapter.
2. Build your care team. Enlist providers who can help you manage the disease. As noted earlier, this team is likely to include a family doctor, as well as others such as a specialist in your chronic disease, a nutritionist, a physiotherapist, and a pharmacist—all would be important members of the team for any of these diseases.
3. Stay abreast of new developments in the treatment of your disease, pharmaceutical or other. Members of the medical community are getting better at treating many of these chronic diseases, as they become both more knowledgeable and more successful in managing the conditions. Do not presume that once you've been diagnosed and a course of treatment has been settled on that this is as good as it gets. You may be able to do better with intensive effort—for example, a combination of medications, diet, and exercise rather than just medications.
4. Introduce adjustments to your life that allow you to more successfully manage your disease—whether it is managing the quality of air in your environment, choosing where you vacation, or avoiding those circumstances that make a disease more difficult to manage. For example, Toronto in

the summertime is not a good place for asthmatics. Plan your life in a way that lets you successfully manage the disease rather than letting a disease manage you.

5. Research the evidence that supports alternatives to long-term medications. Many medications have side effects and consequences, particularly over the longer term. If exercise and a change of diet can spare you from severe symptoms of chronic disease and a lifetime of medication, it is well worth exploring that route, but be sure of the evidence.

Managing Diabetes

> Canada has a diabetes epidemic. More than 2 million Canadians have diabetes today and it's projected to be over 3 million by 2010. This projection is an investment in light of the tripling of overweight and obese children and youth in the last ten years and the aging of our baby boomers. First Nations, Inuit and Métis people as well as new Canadians from high risk countries also face substantial growth in the numbers affected.

The report from which this paragraph is taken goes on to point out the impacts on the Canadian health care system and the economy. "The direct cost to all Canadians for treating diabetes in our hospitals and health care systems is projected to increase 76% by 2016. The indirect economic impact of diabetes on the Canadian economy will also grow. Today, the impact of diabetes on our overall economy is estimated at 13.2 billion dollars," the Canadian Diabetes Association and Diabète Québec said.

In the previous chapter, we looked at ways to prevent diabetes, but even if you have the disease, you shouldn't ignore the tips for prevention. Good eating habits and regular exercise are keystones to maintaining your health. You can also count on the support of your medical team and specialized organizations.

You can live a much better life with diabetes if you tightly manage it. There is assistance, albeit uneven assistance, across Canada to help you with that management challenge. In 2005, the Canadian Diabetes Association and Diabète Québec conducted a survey of members (people who had the disease) that revealed the startling information that only 25 percent of national members and 5 percent of provincial members were aware of any federal or provincial or territorial financial assistance programs to help them manage their diabetes. It's important to know what support is available to you and what the implications of that support can be.

Many people living with diabetes do not have their disease under control. For example, a study has shown that among people living with diabetes for 15 years or more, 62 percent did not have their blood glucose under control. Sixty-three percent of those in the study had high blood pressure, 59 percent had high cholesterol, and 38 percent had micro-vascular foot disease or neuropathy. In short, millions of Canadians with diabetes are not doing a terrific job of managing their disease. A number of provinces—Alberta, Saskatchewan, Ontario, Manitoba, Nova Scotia, and Prince Edward Island—have put strategies in place to prevent and treat diabetes. It is important to know about these strategies and how they can help you. For example, there are 108 Quebec diabetes centres offering diabetes education without requiring a reference from a physician. You can go directly to them.

Paying the Costs

Many Canadians with diabetes are not getting the financial support they deserve and many more are not getting the financial assistance that is already available. The Canadian Diabetes Association provides an example of how financial aid can vary dramatically across the country. They describe Janet, a 22-year-old woman with type 1 diabetes. She has an annual income of about $15,000; she has no private health plan, and relies solely on assistance from the federal and provincial governments. She needs four injections of insulin a day and needs to track her blood glucose levels with strips and a meter. Stunningly, the cost to Janet would vary greatly based on where she lived.

- If she lived in Nunavut, her cost would be zero; the government would pay the entire cost.
- In the Yukon, the cost would be $250 a year, or 1.7 percent of her income.

- In Manitoba, the cost would be $336.40, or 2.3 percent of her income.
- In British Columbia, the cost would be marginally more—$395.85, or 2.7 percent of her income.
- If Janet were living in Ontario or Quebec, she would be spending nearly $950, or 6.6 percent of her income.
- In the birthplace of medicare—Saskatchewan—Janet would need to devote fully 10 percent of her income, or $1451, to cover her medications and supplies.
- In wealthy Alberta, Janet's out-of-pocket costs would be 16.3 percent of her income, or $2359 per year.
- In the four Atlantic provinces, the total costs would run from just over $3000 in Prince Edward Island to over $3600 per year in Newfoundland and Labrador, or almost 25 percent of Janet's income.

Clearly, this is highly inequitable.

The Canadian Diabetes Association's website provides details on the coverage you are eligible for. In addition, you can review information in Chapter 5, "Navigating Your Benefits Plans," to see if there is help for you. If you are working and are part of an employer's health plan, you are likely covered for a pre-existing condition. If you are self-employed or are a student no longer covered under your parents' plan, or for some other reason do not have access to an employer's plan, you will face more difficulty in getting financial aid. However, for more information either visit the Canadian Diabetes

Association's website (www.diabetes.ca) and click on "Programs and Services" or phone your regional office. Your doctor will have contact information for your closest office.

Building a Support Network

Most chronic disease sufferers benefit from a support network. The people who make up this network will be invaluable in helping you navigate the health system. As usual, you start with your family doctor, who may put you in touch with the following professionals:

- Dietitians
- Nurses
- Diabetes educators
- Social workers

In the event that your physician does not have access to a referral network you will need to seek out some or all of the above expertise yourself.

Managing Arthritis

Arthritis is a chronic condition that will affect one in seven Canadians. The most common form is osteoarthritis, which usually affects hips, knees, hands, and spine. It is the leading cause of long-term disability in Canada, and your chance of getting osteoarthritis increases with age. Without effective treatment, arthritis can destroy your joints.

Your first stop as someone recently diagnosed with arthritis should be the website of the Canadian Arthritis Society (www.arthritis.ca). If you prefer, ask your doctor to direct you to the society's nearest office. The website is full of authoritative and peer-reviewed material, as well as chat rooms (gathered together under the heading "Open Forum Community"). When Dennis Morris was leading the Canadian Arthritis Society in the 1990s, he embarked on a project to dramatically improve the website. This was before many other disease-specific groups had started to provide first-class information to members of their association and sufferers of the disease. Morris, a visionary in this respect, recognized the power of information in assisting in the management of chronic disease. Under his stewardship, 10,000 pages of peer-reviewed material on arthritis were placed on the website. The process of peer review—that is, a review by experts knowledgeable in the field of arthritis—guarantees that someone using the website won't be directed to some snake-oil remedy. Unfortunately, many other websites pertaining to health on the Internet look scientific and credible but mask the true ownership and motivation. Often disease-specific websites are designed to sell a particular drug or other miracle cure that may or may not be efficacious. The virtue of the Canadian Arthritis Society's approach was that all the information could be trusted. In addition to the peer-reviewed information, the CAS also provided chat rooms so that arthritis sufferers could communicate with each other about their experiences with particular drugs and other approaches to managing the disease. A second chat room on the site enables those providing care in one part of the country to talk to specialist physicians in another part of the country.

The CAS has provided the Arthritis Self-Management Program (ASMP) for the past decade. This program, offered across Canada, is open to those with arthritis as well as support persons, be they family members or friends. The ASMP deals with issues from exercising with arthritis to eating healthy to protecting joints. More information is available at www.arthritis.ca; click on "Programs and Resources." There is a small charge for the program.

Managing arthritis means managing pain; finding methods of getting daily tasks done, such as getting dressed, cleaning the house, and so on; exercising sensibly (you might think this is the last thing you should do, but in fact a properly designed exercise plan will help you feel much better); and eating well (if you find that certain foods seem to bother you, stay away from them, but be sure to replace any nutrients they may have been providing with something else equally beneficial).

Tip

Movement can actually improve your joints, rather than harming them. Set in place a realistic exercise program with the help of a specialist—then stick to it!

Given that arthritis is a disease with many variations and many degrees of severity, information is a precious commodity. The range of treatments available and their relative success or lack of success in various instances is something that someone living with arthritis especially needs to know. Also valuable is knowledge of new developments in the field of arthritis treatment and centres of expertise.

Paying the Costs

The major cost of treatment for arthritis is for medications. Two categories of non-steroidal anti-inflammatory drugs (NSAIDs) form the basis of care. These are the conventional NSAIDs and the more recently developed COX-2 inhibitors. Newer biologics are entering the market at a very high cost compared to the earlier treatments. The annual cost of treatment with infliximab (Remicade) is estimated to be $12,500 (USD) for the drugs and $18,000 (USD) in total.

These NSAID drugs are covered unevenly across Canada. For persons over the age of 65, there is relatively broad coverage for these classes of medications from public plans. This is less true in Atlantic Canada. For those under the age of 65, coverage depends on the combination of employer plans and public drug programs. If you are with a large, unionized employer, your coverage is likely to be quite comprehensive. Many smaller employers are unable to provide any drug coverage at all for their employees. Again, the situation is best in Quebec and Ontario and worst in Atlantic Canada.

Building a Support Network

The self-management course mentioned earlier is the best starting point. Your support network depends on the severity of your arthritis, but it will require your doctor and your pharmacist. As the disease progresses, you may need other professional health expertise. The self-management program and the chat room on the Canadian Arthritis Society website can be important sources of information. Many patients share their experience with new medications and treatment approaches through the chat room.

By building a solid support network, you can learn to live with arthritis. As usual, your doctor will be your starting point.

Managing Asthma

There is a truly alarming rise in respiratory illnesses, specifically asthma, among children. A generation ago, only a very small percentage of children were diagnosed with asthma, but the number skyrocketed to 12 percent in 2005 for children 12 to 19. The major reason for the rise in asthma is generally believed to be the deterioration in the quality of air we are breathing. In fact, the Ontario Medical Association estimates that bad air causes 5800 avoidable deaths per year in Ontario due to respiratory diseases. They further estimate that 60,000 people visited hospital emergency departments because of the combination of bad air and their underlying asthmatic or respiratory condition. While there is no universal agreement on this data, the trend is unmistakable.

Asthma is chronic inflammation of the lining of the airways of the lungs. It makes these airways contract easily. This in turn makes breathing difficult. There is no cure, but there are techniques and medications for reducing the impact.

Managing asthma is a matter of having a good physician and a good knowledge of what triggers episodes—are you allergic to cats, for example? Does this mean family events should be organized at a cat-free home? To help you cope with your asthma, your family doctor is likely to prescribe two types of drugs that are self-administered through an inhaler. One type is a controller (or preventer), which reduces inflammation. It is normally a medication taken every day. The second type is a reliever, taken to alleviate immediate symptoms.

Paying the Costs

The costs of the drugs and the inhaler are covered unevenly by provincial and employer drug plans. You need to check to see if your provincial government or your employer plan covers the cost of your medications. In all areas of Canada, visits to your family doctor or a specialist for asthma care are covered by provincial plans.

Tip

The Asthma Society of Canada has a useful website with information on asthma and other respiratory diseases. Go to www.asthma.ca. As the Asthma Society notes, your doctor and your asthma educator can do a lot to help you control your symptoms, but there is a lot you can do on your own.

Building a Support Network

The Canadian Asthma Society website offers a very useful tool that allows you to develop your own action plan to manage your condition (click on "Taking Control," then choose "Asthma Action Plan"). The Asthma Action Plan is a strategy to manage your asthma when it gets out of control. One strategy you can try is to make a written agreement with your doctor, as this has been found to improve self-management. The website provides a template you can download to take with you for a discussion with your doctor. Your goal is to have total control, with no daytime or nighttime symptoms; no need to use reliever medication more than four times a week; normal breathing; and no asthma-related school or work absenteeism. When you meet these goals, you are considered to be in the green zone. The yellow zone is where you need to take remedial action, and the red zone is where you must get immediate medical attention. You need to find a way to stay in the green zone and to recognize when you are straying out of it and take action.

Managing Chronic Heart Disease

As noted above, the prevalence of heart disease is broad and expanding. In 1999, 17.4 percent of Canadians over the age of 65 reported having heart disease and 35 percent reported hypertension, a precursor to the disease. Heart disease can be present either after a heart attack or simply with symptoms such as shortness of breath or angina (chest pain). Tens of thousands of Canadians have undergone cardiac rehabilitation, a program of exercise, education, and counselling to help them recover from a heart attack.

Even though millions of Canadians engage in physical activity and diet changes to prevent a future heart attack, not enough of them are choosing a healthy lifestyle. The bad news about the boomer generation is that they are heavier, less fit, and—worse still—in denial about the link between their lifestyle and heart disease. According to a survey by the Heart and Stroke Foundation of Canada, 58 percent of Canadian adults surveyed believe their weight has little or no effect on their heart health. Eighty percent believe that life expectancy will continue to increase. In stark contrast, 50 percent report a sedentary lifestyle, 30 percent are obese, and 21 percent of boomers still smoke. These are much higher risk factors than today's seniors are experiencing—only 11 percent of seniors smoke and only 24 percent are obese. Boomers have high expectations of their health, despite the evidence that their lifestyle puts their heart health at risk. This is despite the reality that

1.3 million Canadian boomers (between 45 and 59) have already been diagnosed with heart disease, stroke, or high blood pressure.

You will likely be prescribed medications to help control your chronic heart disease, but you should also investigate how diet and exercise can aid in improving your health. You may have gathered by now that we're keen on diet and exercise—but we're not alone in knowing that these are fundamental underpinnings to good health. And the heart is one of the most important organs to look after. Any change in diet or physical activity should be undertaken with the full knowledge and advice of your doctor, and this is especially true in the case of those with chronic heart disease.

Paying the Costs

As with other aspects of health care, doctor visits and hospital costs are well covered. Costs for heart medications are largely covered, although there are gaps, as for other medications. It can also take a long time for new medications approved for use in Canada by the federal government and even longer for provincial governments to determine whether patients will be reimbursed. As discussed in depth in Chapters 5 and 6, tax deductions and credits are available for those with heavy medical expenses that are not covered and for those who have resultant disabilities. A new tax credit has been introduced that may assist with costs of fitness and health club memberships.

Building a Support Network

As with other chronic disease, your first stops are your family doctor and the website of the disease-specific organization, in this instance the Heart and Stroke Foundation (at www.heartandstroke.ca). Your team may expand beyond your family doctor to include a cardiologist if you have symptoms other than high blood pressure. If the disease becomes severe, you may be a candidate for one or more heart surgery procedures, ranging from cardiac catheterization, which cleans arteries of plaque, to the insertion of a stent to keep an artery open, to cardiac bypass surgery, which grafts new vessels onto your heart. Over 40,000 Canadians experienced a hospital stay for a heart surgery or procedure in 2000–2001. Many thousands more had procedures or heart diagnostics, such as stress tests, on an outpatient basis.

Most centres of cardiac care expertise are located in the large teaching hospitals that exist across Canada. Often these centres offer information and education as well as services. Two centres are the new Mazankowski Alberta Heart Institute in Edmonton, a part of Capital Health, and the Peter Munk Centre at the Toronto General Hospital, a part of Toronto's University Health Network. Ontario's Cardiac Care Network is an example of how expertise in cardiac care can be linked across sites, as we noted earlier.

Your team may include dietitians and exercise consultants, as well as your pharmacist. It will certainly include a cardiologist.

Managing Mental Illness

We are including mental illness in our discussion of chronic disease, because it's possible that it's the number-one cause of employee absenteeism in Canadian workplaces. Because it's a hidden condition, no one really can measure the depth and breadth of its effects, though we know that more than 4000 Canadians commit suicide a year, and that 1 percent of Canadian families are touched by schizophrenia in some way. A Senate committee chaired by Senator Mike Kirby studied mental illness in Canada and issued its report, *Out of the Shadows—At Last*, in May 2006. The report paints a chilling picture of the challenges faced by Canada's mentally ill. In St. John's, Newfoundland, the Senate committee heard testimony from a young woman who described her long and painful battle with depression. She told of her complete abandonment by and isolation from family and friends, and concluded her testimony by declaring that she wished her illness had been breast cancer rather than depression.

Because mental illness exists in the shadows, as suggested by the report's title, it is a challenging chronic condition to manage. Illnesses such as Alzheimer's disease and other related dementias, while tragic and heartbreaking for the families, are easier to diagnose. But mental illness carries a stigma, and the sufferers work hard to hide their condition. They often manage it by hiding it. If you or someone close to you suffers from mental illness, the section below on building a support network will point you in the right direction to take those first steps to help.

Paying the Costs

We have a mixed system for dealing with mental illness in Canada. Visits to psychiatrists are insured under medicare and paid for by your provincial health insurance. Also covered by medicare are stays in acute care or psychiatric hospitals. Visits to your family doctor, where most mental illness is dealt with in the health system, are also fully insured. However, the coverage for visits to psychologists, therapists, or other mental health professionals is not universal or public. It will rest on the existence and comprehensiveness of your employer plan.

Coverage for medications for various mental illnesses such as depression and bipolar disorder is also fragmented. If you are over 65 or live in Ontario or Quebec, you have broad coverage. If you live in Atlantic Canada, your coverage is comprehensive only during your hospital stay.

The major burden of mental illness in the working-age population falls upon families, owing to lost income. In many instances, employer disability plans can support some of this burden. In other cases, workers' compensation may be able to assist. Often the stigma associated with mental illness is a barrier to exploring all the available supports. This barrier needs to be overcome if the available support, fragmented though it may be, is to be fully accessed.

Building a Support Network

The Canadian Mental Health Association is a fabulous resource. From its website—www.cmha.ca—you can learn about the range of mental illnesses, from mood and eating disorders to schizophrenia and depression. You can also locate the local branch of CMHA in your community. There are also disease-specific societies focused on individual mental illnesses, such as the Schizophrenia Society of Canada (www.schizophrenia.ca) or the Mood Disorders Society of Canada (www.mooddisorders canada.ca).

Members of your support team may include your pharmacist, a psychiatrist, a social worker, and various other therapists, such as a psychologist.

Innovation Across Canada

Across Canada we can find remarkable examples of excellence in chronic disease management. Below is a list of these centres of excellence, with contact information. If you have an opportunity to be served by one of these programs, take advantage what it has to offer. Even if you don't live near one of these programs, you may be able to access information about the program and share it with the providers in your community in the hope that they move in that direction.

DIABETES

Group Health Centre
240 McNabb Street
Sault Ste. Marie, ON P6B 1Y5
Telephone: (705) 759-1234
Fax: (705) 759-7469
www.ghc.on.ca

The Leader Diabetes Initiative, Cypress Region
429 4th Avenue NE
Swift Current, SK S9H 2J9
Telephone: (306) 778-5100
Fax: (306) 773-9513
www.cypresshealth.ca

CHRONIC CARE

Comprehensive Chronic Care, Calgary Region
Macleod Place 1
5920 Macleod Trail SE
Calgary, Alberta T2H 0K2
Telephone: (403) 943-2584
www.calgaryhealthregion.ca

Chronic Disease, Pharmacare and Extended Health Care
www.hss.gov.yk.ca/programs/social_services/disabilities/health_services/

Yukon Health and Social Services
Insured Health Services
4th Floor, Financial Plaza
204 Lambert Street
Whitehorse, Yukon
Telephone: (867) 667-5209

RESOURCE GUIDE

BOOKS

Arthritis Helpbook, 5th Edition. Kate Lorig and James F. Fries (New York: Perseus Books, 2000).

Kate Lorig directs the Arthritis Self-Management Patient Education Project at the Stanford University Arthritis Centre. This is a thorough and practical guide to depending less on medication and more on diet and exercise.

Saving Lives, Saving Money, Transforming Health and Healthcare. Newt Gingrich, with Dana Pavey and Anne Woodbury (Washington, D.C.: The Alexis de Tocqueville Institution, 2003).

For those who came to detest (or even admire) Newt Gingrich during his time as Republican Speaker of the U.S. House of Representatives, this book will be a surprising and positive read. Gingrich has big ideas and offers a range of American examples of excellence in health and health care. In particular, the description of diabetes management in Chapter 8 is an exceptional and direct piece of writing. Newt Gingrich and Hillary Clinton have emerged as the odd couple of American politics—both advocating electronic health records.

WEBSITES FOR DISEASE-SPECIFIC ASSOCIATIONS

Alzheimer Society of Canada: www.alzheimer.ca
The Arthritis Society: www.arthritis.ca
Asthma Society of Canada: www.asthma.ca
Canadian Cancer Society: www.cancer.ca
Canadian Diabetes Association: www.diabetes.ca
Canadian Rheumatology Association: www.rheum.ca
Heart and Stroke Foundation: www.heartandstroke.ca
The Lung Association: www.lung.ca
Multiple Sclerosis Society of Canada: www.mssociety.ca
National Emphysema Foundation: www.emphysemafoundation.org
Parkinson Society of Canada: www.parkinson.ca

OTHER WEBSITES

www.mentalhealthcommission.ca
The Mental Health Commission of Canada, funded by the government of Canada, is an arm's length agency created to focus national attention on mental health issues and to work to improve the health and social outcomes of people living with mental illness.

www.partnershipagainstcancer.ca
The Canadian Partnership Against Cancer is a new, independent, arm's length corporation funded by the government of Canada and charged with accelerating action on cancer control across Canada.

www.publichealth.gc.ca
The Canadian Health Network provides a portal to many of the organizations listed above, as well as to other organizations.

www.healthyontario.com
This terrific website offers information and tips on chronic disease, including a Diabetes Self-Management Centre with advice, videos, and a wealth of useful information.

www.chapters.indigo.ca
The Indigo website has an up-to-date and changing list of health books that the stores carry. See "Books" on the top left, "From Our Trusted Advisors" down the column to the left, then "General Health" and "Healthy Living."

www.keyporter.com
Key Porter Books has published many excellent books on specific chronic diseases. The company's catalogue can be found on-line at the above address or choose "Health and Fitness" from the "Categories" button.

NINE

Coping with Cancer

In 2006, 153,000 Canadians were expected to be diagnosed with cancer. Cancer is primarily a disease of the elderly, with 60 percent of deaths occurring in those 70 years or older.

At least half of all cancers are preventable, and a significant number of the cancers diagnosed are treatable and have excellent survival prospects. In some types of cancer, such as thyroid, the five-year survival rate is very high. For other types, such as late-stage lung cancer, five-year survival rates are not very good.

There are two aspects to navigating the world of cancer treatments and care. Knowing your risk factors is the first. Clearly, none of us wants to develop cancer. Prevention is always the best strategy. The second aspect is navigating the care system if you are diagnosed with cancer. Let's review both aspects, as well as the intermediate ground of screening and early diagnosis.

Prevention: How to Reduce Your Own Cancer Risk

Make sure that you do everything you possibly can to avoid becoming one of those Canadians coping with cancer. You want to reduce your risk of developing any form of cancer. How do you go about it? Fortunately, there is no end of information and advice. One of the

Making a Difference—The Canadian Cancer Control Strategy

In 1999, the Canadian Cancer Society and a number of other cancer organizations banded together to create the Cancer Advocacy Coalition of Canada and to develop a cancer control strategy. The strategy had at its heart risk analysis. Using elaborate, complex, and credible mathematical models, the coalition partners were able to forecast the future of cancer in Canada; they predicted that over the next 40 years Canada would experience 5.9 million new cases. But if the cancer control strategy they proposed were implemented, there would be 1.24 million fewer cases of cancer over 30 years, and the death toll would drop by 423,000. The 2006 federal budget committed $52 million per year for five years to fund the strategy, and work has already started on it. This is good news for Canadians. Avoiding 1.24 million cancer cases over the next 30 years will save not only lives but also a great deal of medical costs. Most important, it will eliminate much pain and suffering for Canadians with cancer and those who care about them. The broad strategy should be of interest to you and should be something you support. The Canadian Cancer Strategy can be found at www.cancer.ca. The coalition of cancer organizations supporting the strategy can be found at www.canceradvocacy.ca.

best sources of information is the Canadian Cancer Society (www.cancer.ca), and much of the information in this chapter is based on materials they produce. The society has suggested taking the following steps to cut down your risk of cancer—at least half of all cancers can be prevented by following these suggestions.

1. Don't start smoking. If you are a smoker, enrol in a stop-smoking program. Avoid second-hand smoke. About 30 percent of all cancer deaths in Canada are attributable to smoking. Cancers associated with smoking can develop in the lungs (lung cancer is the leading cause of death for men and women across Canada), mouth, throat, larynx, cervix, pancreas, esophagus, colon, rectum, kidneys, and bladder. Exposure to second-hand smoke puts non-smokers at higher risk of getting cancer and other lung diseases. Health Canada estimates that more than 300 non-smokers die from lung cancer each year because of second-hand smoke.
2. Eat 5 to 10 servings of fruit and vegetables a day. Choose high-fibre, lower-fat foods. Research suggests that as much as one-third of all cancers are related to what we eat and drink. For a healthy diet, balance your daily meals with foods from the four food groups described in *Canada's Food Guide to Healthy Eating*. Introduce a lot of fibre and dark green leafy vegetables into your diet. If you drink alcohol, limit your intake to one to two drinks

a day. Having one or more alcoholic drinks a day is associated with a slight increase in breast cancer risk. If you are pregnant or breastfeeding, avoid alcohol.

3. Be physically active on a regular basis: This will also help you maintain a healthy body weight. Studies strongly suggest that exercise reduces your risk of colon cancer. Also, the evidence of a link between physical activity and breast cancer is convincing.
4. Protect yourself and your family from the sun. Reduce sun exposure between 11 A.M. and 4 P.M. Seek shade or create your own. Keep babies under one year old out of direct sun. Tanning parlours and sunlamps are not safe. When you are in the sun, always remember SLIP, SLAP, SLOP:
   - SLIP on clothing to cover your arms and legs
   - SLAP on a wide-brimmed hat
   - SLOP on sunscreen (SPF 15 or higher)

   Skin cancer is the most frequently diagnosed cancer in Canada. Check your skin regularly and report any changes to your doctor.
5. Follow cancer-screening guidelines.
   - For women, discuss mammography, Pap tests, and breast exams with a health professional.
   - For men, discuss testicular exams and prostate screening with a health professional.
   - Both men and women should also discuss screening for colon and rectal cancers.

Even people with healthy lifestyles can develop cancer. One way to detect cancer early is to have regular screening tests. These tests can often find cancer when it is still at an early stage. The earlier the cancer is found, the more successful the treatment is likely to be. Screening tests are offered unevenly across the country, although mammograms are more frequently available on an organized and insured basis than either colorectal cancer screening or PSA testing for prostate cancer. In some instances, you may need to pay for a diagnostic test.

6. Visit your doctor or dentist if you notice any change in your normal state of health. Know your body and report any changes (for example, sores that do not heal, a cough that goes on for more than two weeks, or a change in bowel habits) to your doctor or dentist as soon as possible. Health care professionals are trained to spot the early warning signs of cancer and other diseases.
7. Follow health and safety instructions at home and at work when using, storing, and disposing of hazardous materials, household pesticides, or any other chemicals.

Early Detection: Screening and Diagnostic Tests

There are many varieties of cancer, and a number of them are safely and effectively treated if they are detected early.

Taking Steps

The original Canadian Cancer Society plan to reduce risk had six steps. Now it has seven.

In early 2006, Wendy Mesley, a nationally known journalist with the CBC, contracted breast cancer. She went through treatment and returned to the air, having regained her health. However, she was deeply angry about her cancer, since she had followed the original six steps and still contracted the disease. In a documentary she narrated and produced, she asked some very important questions, such as how many cancers are caused by environmental carcinogens or contaminants. The current view of those leading the charge against cancer is that about 10 percent of cancers are environmentally caused, but they readily admit that we know very little about the complex chemistry that sees thousands of new chemicals entering our environment each year. In addition to environmental causes, there are genetic predispositions to certain types of cancer. We have many miles to go on the cancer issue, but the Canadian Cancer Society took an important step by acknowledging that environmental factors are a risk to be avoided.

Michael had a brush with skin cancer over 20 years ago when he noticed a spot on his nose that refused to heal. The spot continued to bleed. Eventually a doctor referred him to a specialist, who diagnosed it as single-cell basal cancer that needed to be surgically removed. Fortunately, he has had no recurrence since. In addition to certain types of skin cancer, colorectal cancers, breast cancer, and thyroid cancer can often be effectively treated if diagnosed early. In fact, patients with thyroid cancer have an almost 98 percent survival five years after surgical intervention. Sadly, there are also dreadful cancers, particularly those later-stage cancers of the lung. Cancers like these are hard, if not impossible, to treat.

How can cancer be detected early? There are three avenues of early detection: population screening, routine testing, and self-examination. Population-based screening tests specific groups, such as women over 50, who should have a mammogram every one to two years to screen for breast cancer. Here are some tests that should be done routinely. If your family doctor doesn't offer them or suggest them, you should request that they be done.

- Pap test: One of the most effective screening tests for cancer of the cervix is the Pap test. Yet many women do not receive a Pap test when they should. It is a simple procedure that can be done in the doctor's office. It takes only a few minutes. It is covered by medicare and should be done every year once a woman becomes sexually active.
- Mammograms: Mammograms are a test for detecting breast cancer before symptoms appear. If you are over the age of 50 and under 69, or if someone in your family had cancer, you should have a mammogram every one to two years. Mammograms are not recommended for women over the age of 69. The test is covered by medicare and is done in a hospital or clinic; it takes only a few minutes. Breast self-examination is another method of detection. However, it will not detect a cancer until it is much larger than one that can be detected by a mammogram.

- Colonoscopy: Both men and women are susceptible to colorectal cancer, which can be detected with a variety of screening tests. One is a colonoscopy, which involves a rectal examination with a scope; for this reason many people resist having this test. It also involves drinking a laxative to clean your colon in preparation for the test. To help alleviate the anxiety you may feel about having this test, you will be given a drug to relax you. The examination takes about 30 minutes. It is conducted in a clinic or hospital. Screening should start when you are over the age of 50. Of the over 8000 people who die of colorectal cancer annually in Canada, nearly all the deaths are unnecessary. Diagnosed early, colorectal cancer has a survival rate approaching 90 percent. Survival falls to 10 percent when it is diagnosed in the later stages. We can't think of more compelling argument for having this simple test.
- FOBT (fecal occult blood test): This test checks for hidden blood in stool samples. Samples are collected at home and sent to a lab, where they are examined. FOBT is the only screening method proven in trials to reduce colorectal cancer deaths. A major pilot project is currently underway in Ontario.
- PSA test: The only available test for prostate cancer has significant accuracy problems. The dilemma is a high rate of both false positives and false negatives. In plain language, the PSA test may miss the disease or indicate that you have it when you don't. Because of

concerns for its accuracy, it is not covered by all provincial governments, although it is widely used.

> **Tip**
>
> Ask your oncologist or other medical specialist to fully explain the accuracy of your PSA result.

- Flexible sigmoidoscopy: This is a scoping examination for colorectal cancer much like a colonoscopy but less extensive. With "flex sig," only the rectum and lower colon are examined.

It's important to know how to manage your diseases and conditions, but you also need to know about managing your health. Tests are only part of that management picture. Two important steps can assist early detection. The first is to find out about your family history, something we mentioned earlier. As some portion of cancer is genetic, you need to know whether family members have had one form of cancer or another. You need to share this information with your doctor, as it will lead to screening at an earlier age for some types of cancer. Second, you need to be alert for warnings from your own body. In Michael's case, the skin lesion that did not heal was the warning signal. Other changes can be visible, like the change of colour of a mole or other skin alterations. The appearance of lumps in a breast found through self-examination or blood in places it shouldn't be are further visible warning signs.

Each type or site of cancer has different screening and diagnostic tests. For example, mammography is used to screen for breast cancer, while biopsies and pathology are used to diagnose it. Pap tests are the means of diagnosing cervical cancer. As noted above, three screening and diagnostics are utilized in colorectal cancer: FOBT (fecal occult blood testing), sigmoidoscopy, and colonoscopy.

Some tests are used for both screening and diagnosis, others for one or the other. The vast majority of people screened do not have cancer. Even those referred after screening for further diagnostic tests may not have cancer. For example, blood detected in an FOBT will likely trigger a colonoscopy, but there are a number of reasons for a positive FOBT that are not cancer. Once you are in the diagnostic/testing process, you may have several tests before a diagnosis is confirmed. Other modalities may be employed, such as ultrasound, X-ray, magnetic resonance imaging (MRI), CAT scan, or even PET scan (in the case of suspected brain cancer).

Tip

Do not fall prey to the fear that more testing is evidence of cancer. Often your doctor is using tests to eliminate possible diagnoses as well as to confirm one.

Getting Your Test Results

There is that moment when your doctor says, "You have cancer." The floor seems to fall out from under you. Few patients accurately remember what is said next. You may be told that your particular type of cancer has a 90 percent survival rate and still go home believing you have been handed a death sentence.

Tips

Do not go alone to hear the test results. Try to take with you someone who listens carefully.

Take pen and paper with you when you go to the doctor. Write down what you are told or ask your companion to take notes.

If you have cancer, you may want to have a special notebook that you take with you everywhere to track your tests and treatments. If you are told you have cancer, ask who will become involved in your care.

Ask what the next steps are.

Ask what the treatment options are.

Get clarity on who to call for help with pain and symptom management. Do you call your family doctor? Your oncologist? Your surgeon or his or her nurse?

Your Team

In the early stages of your cancer care journey and prior to a diagnosis, your family doctor will direct your testing. He or she will then refer you to the relevant specialist. That specialist may be an oncologist or a radiologist. You may also be referred to a specialty centre at a local hospital.

Once a diagnosis is established, your team will likely include an oncologist, a surgeon, and nurses. It's possible a dietitian, home care nurse, social worker, or psychologist will be added to your team if your case is serious and complex.

Tip

If you are battling a difficult cancer that is unresponsive to treatment, one option is to try to enrol in a clinical trial. Before a new drug is approved for use in treating cancer, it must undergo a series of trials. The early trials are to prove that the new drug is safe. Preclinical trials use animals to ensure no risk to humans. The next stage tests the drug on healthy humans to ascertain its safety. Finally, it is used on cancer patients to confirm its efficacy.

The trials you should be interested in are later-stage trials, once the drug has proven its potential. These longer-scale trials are undertaken to establish how the drug compares to other cancer drugs.

Ask your oncologist if you qualify for a clinical trial. If your oncologist is not able to assist, get on the Internet to search for a clinical trial relevant to your type of cancer. Let us be blunt—a clinical trial may provide you with early access to medication capable of extending your life.

In the most simple cases, such as the removal of a small skin cancer, your procedure may be done in an office, clinic, or hospital day surgery. In fact, many cancer surgeries no longer involve an overnight stay. In this case your team will be small. The more complex and longer your cancer journey, the larger your team will become.

Your Treatment

There are three broad categories of treatment for cancer. One is surgical intervention. Some 80 percent of Canadians diagnosed with cancer will have surgery. The second is radiation or radiotherapy treatment. About half of Canadian cancer patients will receive radiation therapy. The third treatment category is drug therapy, generally called chemotherapy or, more recently, systemic therapy. About half of cancer patients will receive systemic therapy.

As you can surmise from the percentages, more than one of these methods may be used in the treatment of cancer. For example, you may have radiation before surgery to shrink the tumour, or you may have radiation after surgery to reduce the chances of reoccurrence. You may have surgery followed by systemic therapy. Treating cancer can be a complex and lengthy business requiring many decisions along the way.

> **Tip**
>
> You need to ask your "next steps" questions persistently to experience the confidence that will help offset some of the stress and fear of your journey. Ask before surgery what would be the indicators for further treatment. Ask when you will know what the next steps in your journey will be.

Cancer Surgery

There is much evidence emerging that where you have cancer surgery is important to your outcome. A number of recent studies have proven the old adage "Practice makes perfect." As a cancer surgery patient you need to understand the practical implications of this statement. All the available data show that higher volumes of surgery are linked to better outcomes. Put differently, hospitals with low volumes of cancer surgery get worse results. How much worse? Consider lung cancer surgery in Ontario. Centres undertaking more than 150 lung cancer surgeries per year have a 30-day mortality rate of 2.42 percent. Those centres doing fewer than 50 surgeries per year have a rate of 3.86 percent. Although that may seem slight, it is actually a 60 percent difference. For the more complex esophagectomy, for cancer of the esophagus, the difference is more dramatic. You have a 10 percent 30-day mortality rate at centres doing seven or fewer procedures per year but only a 1-in-30 rate at centres doing more than 20 procedures per year. A similar variance is found for pancreatic cancer surgery.

The length of stay in hospital for cancer surgery varies a great deal. Many cancer surgeries, like nearly 80 percent of all surgeries, are done on a day-surgery basis. This means no overnight stay in hospital for the patient. You arrive early in the morning and have your surgery. Then, after several hours of recovery and a check to make a certain that all is well, you are discharged home. For more complex cancer surgeries—for colorectal cancer, for example—you are likely to have a hospital stay of four to six days. If there are complications from the surgery, such as an infection, your stay will be longer.

Your care team in the hospital goes well beyond the surgeon. The anaesthetist is a key member of the team, as are the hospital nurses. If your hospital stay is more than one day, you will be cared for by the team on the hospital ward. Your surgeon will visit to check on your progress, recommending when you can eat again, when you can get out of bed, and when you can go home. The nursing team will be supplemented by dietary (food) services and sometimes a specialized pain management team.

Tip

During your stay you may come into contact with as many as 40 or 50 different care providers. Check all major decisions (drug changes, meals) with your surgeon.

To support a patient's recovery at home after surgery, all provinces provide home-care services. These services are arranged through the hospital's discharge planner. The home-care service can include nursing care, homemaker services, pain management, and wound care, depending on patient needs. Basic home-care services are paid by provincial governments. You may wish to purchase supplementary hours privately. Many services are available for an hourly rate.

Tip

Arrange for home-care services before you have your surgery.

Radiation

Radiation therapy, sometimes called radiotherapy or X-ray therapy, is the use of radiation to treat cancer. High doses of radiation kill cancerous cells or keep them from growing. The central problem with radiation therapy is that, despite efforts at protective shielding, it can damage normal cells.

Radiation therapy is often used in combination with surgery. It may be used before surgery to shrink a tumour and allow it to be more easily removed. This type of therapy may also be used to stop cancer cell growth after surgery.

Radiation therapy can be given externally through a linear accelerator—a machine that produces and delivers radiation in a very precise way—or internally through radioactive implanted seeds.

From the patient's perspective, radiation therapy is painless but often accompanied by side effects. The most obvious side effect is hair loss, but others can include fatigue, difficulties eating, and skin irritation. Often patients don't know whom to consult about side effects. By the time of radiation therapy, a patient usually has involved in her treatment her family doctor, a medical oncologist, possibly a surgeon, and the radiation oncology team (which may include a radiation oncologist, radiation physicist, dosimetrist, radiation therapist, and radiation nurse). Her broader team may include a dietitian, social worker, and physical therapist, among others.

Tip

Before starting radiation therapy, get a clear answer to the question "Who do I call about managing side effects?"

Chemotherapy

Chemotherapy is the use of drugs to treat cancer. Often more than one drug is used in a combination chemotherapy. This treatment may be used to cure cancer, to control cancer, or to relieve symptoms (such as pain). Chemotherapy may be given in a variety of ways, including through an intravenous delivery system, orally, or topically—on your skin.

Side effects of chemotherapy can include fatigue, nausea and vomiting, pain, and hair loss. As with radiation therapy, you need to know whom to contact about side effects. You also need support to cope with the stresses and physical incapacity. You need to be alert to signs of infection, such as high fever.

Tip

Chemotherapy can be a very difficult treatment regime. It is wise to discuss both the risks and the benefits before beginning treatment.

Navigating the Cancer Care System

During your treatment, you will experience a wide range of emotions. There will be times when you'll be exhausted and easily overwhelmed by the choices you have to make and just by coping with the new world you've entered. Fortunately, there are agencies whose job is to provide help and information to you. In addition, take advantage of every offer of help from friends, family, and neighbours. Here are some services that should be available to you:

- Through your local Canadian Cancer Society (CCS) branch, you can arrange to be driven to treatments. You need to book ahead, and you may find yourself sharing the vehicle with other cancer patients. Contact information for the CCS is listed at the end of this chapter.
- Some patients and their families will be eligible for home care, as noted earlier. Home care is available through governments in many provinces, through the local health region in others, and in Ontario through Community Care Access Centres.
- Palliative care is a necessity for many cancer patients. Palliative care and supports are covered in Chapter 11, "Navigating End-of-Life Care."
- Advocacy organizations such as the Canadian Cancer Society, which has branches across Canada, are excellent sources of information. Be sure to check out the websites of disease-specific cancer groups, such as lung cancer groups and breast cancer groups, and also those of cancer treatment organizations such as Cancer Care Ontario and the B.C. Cancer Agency.

Provincial Cancer Agencies

Provincial cancer agencies are public organizations that coordinate cancer services and prevention programs. Most provinces have cancer agencies, although the scope and range of their services vary. Some agencies focus on management of radiation therapy while others also include systemic therapies. Although their main focus is treatment, they are also a great source of information.

Tip

The focus of the Canadian Cancer Society is on providing information and support. Other cancer organizations run the gamut from very specific advocacy to research to information.

RESOURCE GUIDE

Your three key resources for your cancer care journey are

- Provincial cancer agencies
- Canadian Cancer Society
- Other cancer organizations

PROVINCIAL CANCER AGENCIES

Alberta

Alberta Cancer Board
Standard Life Centre
10405 Jasper Avenue, Suite 1220
Edmonton, AB T5J 3N4

Telephone: (780) 412-6300
Fax: (780) 412-6326

Cross Cancer Institute
Department of Medical Physics
11560 University Avenue
Edmonton, AB T6G 1Z2
Telephone: (403) 432-8750
Fax: (403) 432-8615

Tom Baker Cancer Centre
Department of Medical Physics
1331–29th Street NW
Calgary, AB T2M 4N2
Telephone: (403) 944-1789
Fax: (403) 944-2327

British Columbia
B.C. Cancer Agency
675 West 10th Avenue
Vancouver, BC V52 1C3
Telephone: (604) 675-8000
Toll-free: 1-800-663-3333
www.bccancer.bc.ca

Manitoba
CancerCare Manitoba
675 McDermot Avenue
Winnipeg, MB R3E 0V9

Telephone: (204) 787-2197
Toll-free: 1-866-561-1026
www.cancercare.mb.ca

New Brunswick
Centre d'Oncologie Dr. L. Richard
Hôpital Dr. Georges-L. Dumont
330 rue Archibald
Moncton, NB E1C 2Z3
Telephone: (506) 862-4151
Fax: (506) 862-4222

Saint John Regional Hospital
Department of Therapeutic Physics
P.O. Box 2100
Saint John, NB E2L 4L2
Telephone: (506) 648-7410
Fax: (506) 648-6880

Newfoundland
Dr. H. Bliss Murphy Cancer Clinic
Department of Medical Physics
300 Prince Philip Drive
St. John's, NL A1B 3V6
Telephone: (709) 777-7589
Fax: (709) 753-0927
www.cancercarefoundation.nl.ca

Nova Scotia
Nova Scotia Cancer Centre
QEII Health Sciences Centre
5820 University Avenue
Halifax, NS B3H 1V9
Telephone: (902) 473-6017
Fax: (902) 473-6120
www.cancercare.ns.ca

Ontario
Cancer Care Ontario/Action Cancer Ontario
620 University Avenue
Toronto, ON M5G 2L7
Telephone: (416) 971-9800
Fax: (416) 971-6888
www.cancercare.on.ca

Prince Edward Island
PEI Cancer Treatment Centre
Queen Elizabeth Hospital
P.O. Box 6600
Charlottetown, PE C1A 8T5
Telephone: (902) 894-2027
www.cancercare.pe.ca

Saskatchewan
Saskatchewan Cancer Agency
Allan Blair Cancer Centre
4101 Dewdney Avenue

Regina, SK S4T 7T1
Telephone: (306) 766-2213
Fax: (306) 766-2688
www.saskcancer.ca

Saskatoon Cancer Centre
20 Campus Drive
Saskatoon, SK S7N 4H4
Telephone: (306) 655-2662
Fax: (306) 655-2910
www.saskcancer.ca

CANADIAN CANCER SOCIETY BRANCHES

Canadian Cancer Society
National Office
10 Alcorn Avenue, Suite 200
Toronto, ON M4V 3B1
Telephone: (416) 961-7223
Fax: (416) 961-4189
www.cancer.ca

Or contact your closest office from the list below:

Alberta Division
325 Manning Road NE, Suite 200
Calgary, AB T2E 2P5
Telephone: (403) 205-3966
Fax: (403) 205-3979

British Columbia and Yukon Division
565 West 10th Avenue
Vancouver, BC V5Z 4J4
E-mail: inquiries@bc.cancer.ca
Telephone: (604) 872-4400
Toll-free: 1-800-663-2524
Fax: (604) 879-4405

Manitoba Division
193 Sherbrook Street
Winnipeg, MB R3C 2B7
E-mail: info@mb.cancer.ca
Telephone: (204) 774-7483
Fax: (204) 774-7500

New Brunswick Division
133 Prince William Street
P.O. Box 2089
Saint John, NB E2L 3T5
E-mail: ccsnb@nb.cancer.ca
Telephone: (506) 634-6272
Fax: (506) 634-3808

Newfoundland and Labrador Division
P.O. Box 8921
Viking Building
St. John's, NL A1B 3R9
E-mail: ccs@nl.cancer.ca

Telephone: (709) 753-6520
Fax: (709) 753-9314

Northwest Territories Unit
5016 - 50 Avenue
P.O. Box 2007
Yellowknife, NT X1A 2P5
Telephone: (867) 920-4428
Fax: (867) 920-4162

Nova Scotia Division
5826 South Street, Suite 1
Halifax, NS B3H 1S6
E-mail: ccs.ns@ns.cancer.ca
Telephone: (902) 423-6183
Fax: (902) 429-6563

Ontario Division
1639 Yonge Street
Toronto, ON M4T 2W6
E-mail: ontdiv@ontario.cancer.ca
Telephone: (416) 488-5400
Fax: (416) 488-2872

Prince Edward Island Division
1 Rochford Street, Suite 1
Charlottetown, PE C1A 9L2
E-mail: info@pei.cancer.ca

Telephone: (902) 566-4007
Fax: (902) 628-8281

Quebec Division
5151 L'Assomption Boulevard
Montreal, QC H1T 4A9
E-mail: webmestre@quebec.cancer.ca
Telephone: (514) 255-5151
Fax: (514) 255-2808

Saskatchewan Division
1910 McIntyre Street
Regina, SK S4P 2R3
E-mail: ccssk@sk.cancer.ca
Telephone: (306) 790-5822
Fax: (306) 569-2133

OTHER CANCER ORGANIZATIONS

Cancer Advocacy Coalition Canada
www.canceradvocacy.ca
As noted at the beginning of this chapter, the coalition is an umbrella group and its website reflects this reality. It is best viewed as a source of links to other information sources.

DISEASE-SPECIFIC SITES

Alliance for Lung Cancer Advocacy, Support and Education: alcase.org

Association of Cancer Online Resources: www.acor.org
Breast Cancer Action Saskatchewan: www.bcask.ca
Breast Cancer Network Nova Scotia: www.bca.ns.ca
Canadian Breast Cancer Foundation: www.cbcf.org
Canadian Breast Cancer Network: www.cbcn.ca
Canadian Breast Cancer Research Alliance: www.breast.cancer.ca
CancerCare: LungCancer.org
CancerNews on the Net: www.cancernews.com
Cancerpage.com (treatment guidelines, news, clinical trials): www.cancerpage.com
CancerWeb: infoventures.com/cancer
Candlelighters Childhood Cancer Foundation: www. candlelighters.org
Early Prostate Cancer Diagnosis Ontario: www.health.gov.on.ca/english/providers/pub/cancer/psa/psa_summary/summary.html
Gilda's Club: www.gildasclub.org
Intercultural Cancer Council: www.iccnetwork.org
Lung Cancer Canada: lungcancercanada.ca
Lymphoma Foundation Canada: www.lymphoma.ca
Malecare, Inc. (prostate, testicular, and male breast cancer): malecare.com
National Alliance of Breast Cancer Organizations (U.S.): http://nabco.org
National Breast Cancer Coalition (U.S.): www.stop breastcancer.org
National Cancer Institute (U.S.): www.cancer.gov

National Cancer Institute's Cancer Information Service: cis.nci.nih.gov

National Ovarian Cancer Organization: www.ovariancanada.org

Ovarian Cancer Canada: www.ovariancancercanada.ca

Prostate cancer information: Procure.ca

Prostate Centre at Vancouver General Hospital: Prostatecentre.com

Prostate Cancer Foundation (U.S.): Prostatecancerfoundation.org

Willow Breast Cancer Support and Resource Services: www.willow.org

World Conference on Breast Cancer Foundation: www.wcbcf.ca

PALLIATIVE CARE

Canadian Hospice Palliative Care Association: www.chpca.net

Choices in Dying: www.compassionandchoices.org

Partners against Pain (U.S.): www.partnersagainstpain.com

CLINICAL TRIALS

National Cancer Institute, Clinical Trials (U.S.): www.cancer.gov/clinicaltrials

Ontario Cancer Research Network, Ontario Cancer Trials: ontariocancertrials.ca

INTERNATIONAL ORGANIZATIONS

The best international site for information is the National Cancer Institute: www.nci.nih.gov

American Cancer Society: www.cancer.org

American Institute for Cancer Research: aicr.org

American Society of Clinical Oncology: www.asco.org

CancerBackup: www.cancerbackup.org.uk

CancerCare (U.S. social service agency providing services to cancer patients and families): cancer care.org

Cancer Index (a guide to Internet resources for cancer): www.cancer-index.org

Cancer Research UK: cancerresearchuk.org

Cancerworld.com: www.cancereurope.org

European Institute of Women's Health, Women's Cancer Information Project: www.eurohealth.ie/cancom

European Society for Medical Oncology: www.esmo.org

Federation of European Cancer Societies: www.ecco-org.eu

Lymphoma Research Foundation of America: www. lymphoma.org

Mayo Clinic Cancer Resource Center: www.mayoclinic. com

National Cancer Institute: www.cancer.gov

National Comprehensive Cancer Network: www.nccn. org

Oncology Nursing Society (U.S.): www.ons.org

Pan American Health Organization: www.paho.org

Patient Advocate Foundation (U.S.): www.patient advocate.org

University of Pennsylvania, Abramson Cancer Center: www.oncolink.com

US TOO International Prostate Cancer Education and Support Network (U.S.): www.ustoo.com

World Health Organization Health for All Database: www.who.dk

MEDICAL JOURNALS

If you want to research your condition, the following journals either are devoted entirely to cancer or frequently include cancer studies. These are technical medical journals, but many articles are surprisingly easy to read. Some local libraries carry copies of these journals. Often you will find that new research results are rapidly reported in the media. The CNN and CBC websites both have health sections.

American Journal of Clinical Oncology: www.amjclinicaloncology.com

Canadian Journal of Oncology (articles from the National Library of Medicine database)

Canadian Medical Association Journal: www.cmaj.ca

Cancer Detection and Prevention: www.cancerprev.org

The Cancer Letter: www.cancerletter.com

Journal of the National Cancer Institute: www.jnci.oupjournals.org

Lancet (UK medical journal): www.thelancet.com

New England Journal of Medicine: content.nejm.org

BOOKS

There are shelves filled with books on coping with cancer in any major bookstore or library. Most are specific to a type of cancer. We're suggesting these very few as being of particular interest.

Foods That Fight Cancer: Preventing and Treating Cancer Through Diet. Richard Beliveau (Toronto: McClelland and Stewart, 2006).

This book by biochemist Richard Beliveau was a sensation in Quebec, where a French version sold 138,000 copies (when 5000 copies is viewed as a bestseller).

Everyone's Guide to Cancer Therapy, Fourth Edition. Malin Dollinger, Ernest Rosenbaum, and Greg Cable (Kansas City: Andrews McMeel Publishing, 2002).

An easy, though lengthy (848 pages), guide to cancer therapies.

Should I Be Tested for Cancer? H. Gilbert Welch (Berkeley: University of California Press, 2004).

A very balanced perspective on the pros and cons of testing for cancer.

Goes Down Easy: Recipes to Help You Cope with the Challenge of Eating During Cancer Treatment. Elise Mecklinger, with the Princess Margaret Hospital Dietitians (2006).

Cookbook author Elise Mecklinger worked closely with a team of six registered dietitians at Toronto's Princess Margaret Hospital to develop the recipes for this book. Inspired by patients' requests for easy, practical recipes to deal with certain nutrition problems while undergoing cancer treatment, the book is a practical guide for people living with cancer, their families, and their caregivers. The recipes are grouped to deal with specific concerns, such as loss of appetite, nausea, changes in taste, sore mouth and swallowing problems, and diarrhea. Proceeds of sales go to the Princess Margaret Hospital Foundation. To order, go to www.pmhf.ca and click on Online Store. Or call 1-866-YES-PMHF or 1-866-937-7643 (toll-free).

Stopping Cancer at the Source. Sara Rosenthal (Trafford and Your Health Press, 2001).

A guide to reducing your risk, as well as a review of environmental risks.

Breast Cancer: Beyond Convention. Mary Tagliaferri, Isaac Cohen, Debu Tripathy (New York: Pocket Books, 2003).

A range of alternative theories are covered in this book.

TEN

Navigating Health Care for Seniors

Today, owing to medical advancements, more and more seniors are living much longer—this group is commonly referred to as the "aging population." Canada's famous demographic expert, Professor David Foot, has filled many lecture halls speaking about the implications of the aging population for Canada.

Although living longer is something we all aspire to, the aging population is certainly a cause for concern because of the health care implications. We know that seniors account for the highest costs to our health care system. In 2003, people over 65 were 12.8 percent of the population, but they racked up 43 percent of provincial health care spending. By 2026, seniors were projected to be 21 percent of the total population. Seniors have more chronic disease and require more medical and pharmaceutical interventions. Some seniors are unable to live by

Aging in Canada: Important Facts

- Seniors (individuals aged 65 and over) constitute the fastest-growing population group in Canada.
- In 2001, it was estimated that 3.92 million Canadians were 65 years of age or older: That figure is two-thirds more than it was in 1981.
- The seniors' population is expected to reach 6.7 million in 2021 and 9.2 million in 2041 (nearly one in four Canadians).
- The growth of the seniors' population will account for close to half of the growth of the overall Canadian population in the next four decades.

Source: Adapted from Health Canada, "Canada's Aging Population" by Insurance Canada; available at www.insurance-canada.ca.

Life Expectancy in Canada: Important Facts

- In 1920, 5 percent of the population was over age 65; by the year 2020, it will be close to 20 percent.
- In 1920, the average Canadian could expect to live to the age of 59. By 1996, a 65-year-old man could expect to live to age 81, and a woman to age 85.
- Close to 30 percent of individuals between the ages of 75 and 84 and 45 percent of those over age 85 have a long-term disability.
- Although women will outlive men by an average of four years, only one of these additional years is expected to be free of disability. Two of the three remaining years are expected to involve severe disability.

Source: Adapted from Statistics Canada by Clarica; available at www.insurance-canada.ca.

themselves and require specialized housing that can accommodate their health care needs.

Rapid growth in the number of seniors, coupled with the longer life expectancy, has serious implications on health care costs for both government and the individual.

Drug Coverage and Seniors

As discussed in Chapter 5, "Navigating Your Benefits Plans," all jurisdictions have some form of provincial drug plan to significantly reduce the cost burden to seniors. However, these plans tend to be a patchwork across the country.

- In Ontario, British Columbia, and Alberta, all residents are automatically covered under relatively generous public drug plans when they turn 65. In these provinces, even seniors who are not considered to be of low income benefit from drug plans for which they pay no premium. Often these plans have either no deductible at all or a modest annual deductible. In these three provinces, most seniors take advantage of the seniors' drug program.
- In the Atlantic provinces, seniors have to either pay very high premiums or satisfy certain high requirements in order to be eligible to benefit from the provincial drug plan.
- In Saskatchewan and Manitoba, provincial drug benefits programs provide a public subsidy to all residents, regardless of age, who have high drug costs

relative to income. Under these programs, income-based deductibles mean many seniors do not receive the public subsidy.

- Quebec has a slightly different system of coverage for seniors. In this province, seniors purchase drug coverage through a government-operated compulsory plan for all those (seniors and non-seniors alike) who do not have a private drug plan through an employer or affinity-group coverage.
- The territories cover seniors over 65 for their medications as long as they are on the territorial formulary. The Yukon covers the total cost of the lowest-price generics of all pharmaceutical medications listed in the Yukon formulary as well as the dispensing fee. However, the program is to be used as the insurer of "last resort," meaning that if a senior has coverage under any other plan, he or she must seek reimbursement elsewhere first. The Northwest Territories covers seniors through Alberta Blue Cross (which administers the plan). Basically seniors get 100 percent coverage on all drugs listed on the territorial formulary.

All provinces (with the exception of Manitoba) expect seniors to pay some portion of the professional (or dispensing) fee of the drug. The dispensing fee is the fee that the pharmacy charges for filling the prescription. It is not the cost of the drug.

Tips

Seek out a pharmacy with low dispensing fees. For example, Wal-Mart currently does not charge a dispensing fee.

Canadian mail-order or on-line pharmacies have low or no dispensing fees and great prices. Mail-order pharmacies do not provide the kind of hand holding and advice that bricks-and-mortar pharmacies do, but they are inexpensive because they do not have much overhead and they will deliver by courier at no charge to you.

Mail-Order or On-line Pharmacies

Canadian pharmacy mail-order services are also accessible on-line. They are licensed to dispense medications and require valid prescriptions from a physician who is licensed in your area. With some services, you can choose the medication on-line (along with the dosage and number of tablets) and pay with a credit card. For your order to be filled, you will need to e-mail, fax, or mail in the written prescription. Some of these services offer the order forms on-line; you fill them out (by browsing the website for the product you need) and fax or mail them in along with the written prescription.

The prescription is the ultimate order form, so if you fill out the order form improperly or don't correctly select the right product or dosage, the pharmacist will be guided by the prescription. These services offer toll-free numbers for help with placing orders.

Mail-order services cannot fill certain prescriptions, such as those for Valium or Tylenol 3, because they are not allowed to ship narcotics in Canada. They also have limits on the number of repeats they can fill at a time. Typically, mail-order services will guarantee delivery within a certain time period, but don't expect next-day delivery. The guarantees tend to be at least two weeks. This is not a practical option for people who need to fill their prescription immediately. However, for chronic conditions that require regular filling of prescriptions, mail-order pharmacies can be great, especially if you normally have to pay for a portion of the drug or portion of the dispensing fee.

What's Covered?

All provincial and territorial plans cover only those medications that are on the formulary that has been approved by the province. Why do some medicines make it on the formulary and others don't? Cost containment is usually the reason.

In Chapter 5, we discussed the issue of generic substitution, but we're going to review it again here. When there are multiple medications (brand-name and generic medications) on the market and the jurisdiction has ruled that these products are virtually the same, it will often allow coverage only on the less expensive generic version. This is called "generic substitution." Once a pharmaceutical company puts a new drug on the market, it has a number of years of patent protection, which guarantees that a copy of that original drug cannot be sold on the market. Once the patent protection expires, however, any company can (and will) produce a copy of the medication. These "copies" are called generic medications and are less expensive than the original brand-name pharmaceutical drug. In many provinces, seniors' drug benefits plans promote substituting brand medications with generic medications. They do this by covering only up to a certain amount (usually the cost of the least expensive product). But if the senior wishes to have the brand-name medication, he or she can pay the difference.

Generic substitution has been the cause of a number of legal and public relations battles among generic and brand drug manufacturers. The brand drug manufacturers argue that while medications may contain the same active ingredients, there can be differences in the way they are administered or the number of daily doses that the patient needs to take. These differences, they argue, are significant, and therefore substitution with another product is not desirable.

Seniors' formularies restrict certain drugs either because they are deemed to be cost effective only under certain circumstances or because there is a high potential for their overuse or misuse. In these cases, seniors will require their doctors to request special authorizations or approvals if they wish to prescribe that particular medication. This practice helps governments ensure that medications are being prescribed for the right reasons.

Many would argue, however, that these restrictions are little more than cost-cutting measures.

Seniors are also eligible for coverage on other things besides drugs, such as dental, eyeglasses, and medical devices. However, once again, each jurisdiction has different levels of coverage, different qualifying rules, different dollar limits, and/or different lengths of time between new purchases of these items. Seniors will need to contact their own jurisdiction to understand the rules of the game and the coverage to which they are entitled.

Managing Multiple Medications

Seniors frequently take numerous medications—on average, those 65 and over take five different medications at a time. It is absolutely crucial for seniors to manage their medications closely. Here are some tips to help with that management

Choose a Home Pharmacy

Decide which pharmacy will be your "home pharmacy" and always go to that pharmacy to fill your medications. By going to the same pharmacy, you will ensure that the pharmacist can track what you are taking and tell you if it reacts to something else you are taking. If for some reason you need to get your prescription filled elsewhere, always go back to your home pharmacy with the new prescription and ask them to record it so that it is registered and the pharmacist can better monitor your medications.

Read the Directions

Always pay very close attention to the directions on *how* to take the medication and not just on *when* to take it. Frequently these directions ensure that the medication is properly absorbed into your body. When a medication is not absorbed properly, it can be like not taking it at all. Some directions include the following:

- Take on an empty stomach.
- Take with food.
- Not to be taken with milk (or other things like minerals).

If you aren't certain if your vitamins contain some of the ingredients that must not be taken within a few hours of your medication, check with the pharmacist (not the doctor). The pharmacist will have a better idea of what vitamins or other medications you will need to avoid.

In addition, some pharmacies provide a printed information sheet about your medication. Read it carefully and keep it on file so it is always handy. These sheets list side effects you can expect. Shoppers Drug Mart's

> **Tip**
>
> If you have to go to the hospital because of an emergency, you will be asked what medications you are taking. In such situations, it can be hard to remember them, even if you are taking only two or three. Keep a list by the phone or in some other easy-to-get-to place so ambulance staff or others can take it along and inform the hospital about your meds.

HealthWatch bulletin, which accompanies all prescriptions, is especially helpful.

Taking the Medications

If your drug plan substitutes one drug for another similar drug, do not assume that the directions and dosage times are the same. The medication may need to be taken at different times and/or differently than the medication you are used to taking. It is essential that you check the directions each time you fill a script.

Tips

Some people like to put their daily or weekly medication doses into a pill box. This is fine, but here are some additional tips that you should follow:

- Make sure that you keep a log of what needs to be taken, what it looks like, and when and how it needs to be taken. The log becomes more important when you use a pill box because you are now removing the pills from the original containers. All the information on the container must be transferred to a daily log or you or a caregiver may get confused.
- If you are looking after an elderly relative or friend who uses a pill box (especially a weekly pill box), make certain you or someone else is helping that person load it up. Many elderly people start to lose coordination or have problems with their memory and accidentally load the medications into the wrong slots.
- Pharmacists can also make up a blister pack that saves the patient the organizational effort. Be sure you or your caregiver can open the blister—sometimes the packaging can be quite tough.

The best way—in fact, the only safe way—to properly manage taking more than one medication is to make a daily schedule and log in what you need to take (even the colour), how it needs to be taken, and when it is to be taken. Usually a one-day schedule is all you need since most medications are taken daily.

Here is an example of a daily log. In this example, the person needs to take two medications with different directions. One medication needs to be taken on an empty stomach twice a day (at least one hour before or two hours after eating). The second medication cannot be taken with any minerals and needs to be taken three times a day:

12:00 am	Medication X (small red pill) can't take with any minerals!
1:00 am	
2:00 am	
3:00 am	
4:00 am	
5:00 am	
6:00 am	Medication Y (blue pill) take on empty stomach 2 X day
7:00 am	Earliest I can have breakfast
8:00 am	Medication X (small red pill) can't take with any minerals!
9:00 am	
12:00 pm	Take my vitamins and minerals no earlier than noon!
	Best time for lunch
1:00 pm	

2:00 pm	
3:00 pm	Do not take my vitamins and minerals after 3!
4:00 pm	Medication X (small red pill) can't take with any minerals!
5:00 pm	
6:00 pm	Medication Y (blue pill) take on empty stomach
7:00 pm	Supper (earliest)
8:00 pm	
9:00 pm	
10:00 pm	
11:00 pm	

Clearly, these are fictitious medications; however, the importance of the log is clear. It not only tracks when medications need to be taken, but also helps a senior plan his or her day around the directions for taking that medication. Without planning in advance, a senior could easily forget that he or she can't eat until a certain time and might end up having a meal too close to taking a medication that only works properly on an empty stomach. Also, when there is a conflict in the schedule, seniors may skip a meal or postpone taking their medication to rectify the problem. None of these situations is good, and all can be easily avoided with a formal day schedule.

Home-Care Services for Seniors

Seniors have different housing needs from younger people and from one another. Most choose to remain at home and require virtually no support, while others will need some support in order to manage their own care. This is often a time of transition for the family and the senior, and it can be an issue that needs to be reviewed from time to time. Sometimes, the family's hand is forced through illness or accident, and they find themselves facing questions about how to maintain the senior's independence, how to ensure safety, and what is best all round for the senior.

All jurisdictions offer some community support for seniors living at home who have been assessed by the appropriate provincial or territorial agency and are deemed to require these services. As with most health services beyond hospitals and doctors, there is little consistency from province to province. You will need to check exactly what your province or territory will provide in home care. All jurisdictions require that a needs assessment be completed in order for you or a loved one to get access to government-covered services. In Ontario, if you are in the hospital, the discharge planner will organize access to home care. If you are not in the hospital, you will need to contact your local Community Care Access Centre (CCAC), and they will conduct an assessment. In provinces that are regionally organized, such as most other provinces in Canada, generally you will need to contact the regional health authority, which will provide a needs assessment and will be able to organize the care and/or support to which you are entitled. The resource section at the end of this chapter provides you with contact information for some of these services—the Seniors Canada site is an especially important one for seniors and their family members to know about.

Across the board, there are four main categories of home- and community-based services for seniors (some are covered in some provinces or territories if you pass the needs assessment and/or the income test):

- *Visiting Health Professional Services.* These services allow seniors to be visited in their own home by a health professional, generally a nurse, for the purpose of assessing and planning to address the seniors' needs, as well as providing home health care.
- *Personal Care and Support.* These services provide support for a variety of daily living activities that include bathing, dressing, and eating.
- *Homemaking.* These services include things like shopping, light housekeeping, and meal preparation.
- *Community Support Services.* These services provide support in areas that include transportation, meal deliveries, social and recreational services, caregiver relief, and security checks.

If you choose to receive home care instead of institutional care, you need to know that home-care services provided by the government vary according to the jurisdiction and the resources available in the community. Government-funded home-care services are typically restricted to a fixed number of hours per week or per month.

You may need to supplement with private care beyond what your province provides. According to Clarica Insurance, a company with experience in private care insurance, the costs for homemaking, personal care, and nursing care can vary from $11 to over $40 per hour, depending on the type of care you need and the costs in your area. The Victorian Order of Nurses (VON) reports that an RN or auxiliary nurse can cost anywhere from $30 to $38 per hour and a medical services aide can cost from $14 to $19 per hour.

The following are some important factors to consider when determining whether to stay at home or pursue residence in a facility such as a nursing home or a retirement home (see below for definitions of these types of accommodation):

1. What are your medical and personal support needs?
2. What do you value or what is important to you?
3. What support can your family or friends provide? This can be important in determining whether you just need a little extra support to remain at home.
4. What does your community, province, regional health authority, or territory provide and what are you eligible for under the publicly funded health care system? The government (in the form of a regional health authority or government agency

like the CCAC in Ontario) usually sets the eligibility criteria for services.

5. What can you afford outside of what is available to you? Getting help from a combination of resources, like publicly funded services, support services from family and friends, and community services (for example, through your municipality or church, synagogue, or mosque), will often provide a fairly cost-effective solution.
6. Remember that there is a fairly high demand for all publicly funded services and that means wait lists can be long. Plan ahead, whether it is for you or for an elderly loved one. Getting access to government-sponsored services can mean waiting months. Clearly, to take advantage of what is available through public funding, you will need to start early to gather information so that when you need to act, often suddenly, you have all the information.

Long-term Care Housing Options for Seniors

There are three basic categories of housing options for seniors:

1. *Supportive Housing*. Supportive housing goes by many names, including assisted living and independent living. This housing is geared to seniors who require minimal to moderate levels of support in order to live independently. Rent is

often geared toward seniors' income levels through the use of subsidies. Though publicly funded services (like home care) can be provided in these homes, the rent and services are paid through subsidies and by the residents.

2. *Retirement Homes.* These homes are privately run rental accommodations for seniors who are able to live independently with a minimum of support. The services offered range from modest to deluxe, and they are exclusively paid for by the residents. Home-care services that are publicly funded and deemed necessary for eligible seniors can be delivered on site in these residences.
3. *Funded Facilities—Nursing Homes or Long-term Care Facilities.* Long-term care facilities are also known throughout Canada as nursing homes. These residences provide housing for seniors who require more support for living and for health care. Licensed nursing homes can be run by for-profit or not-for-profit organizations. Since licensed nursing homes are partially funded, wait times can be long. Note the word "licensed": All nursing homes, whether for profit or not, are inspected and must be licensed. Retirement homes are not licensed.

Applying for a Funded Nursing Home

In every jurisdiction in Canada, you will need to undergo a needs assessment to determine if you are eligible to enter a funded facility based on the type of support or care you need. Naturally, the first big criterion is that you are eligible for medicare (i.e., you have a health card) in Canada. The next step is to contact your regional health authority or provincial or territorial government and ask about seniors' housing—there is no single website to go to. If you live in Ontario, you need to contact your local CCAC. All provincial and territorial governments provide information on their websites about where to call.

Once you have contacted the appropriate government agency, a case manager will be assigned to help you navigate the complexity of the health care system and link you with the right information. These case managers will also organize a needs assessment, which is how they will determine your specific needs. For example, do you have problems with mobility? Do you have family supports in place? Do you have financial difficulties? A case manager can also help determine how to put a number of different community supports in place to best meet your needs. He or she will then be able to prioritize your case. The most urgent cases will be moved up the list.

Funding and Fees

As mentioned above, licensed nursing homes in Canada are partially funded, meaning that they provide 24-hour publicly funded nursing care and health care services to their residents, and in some jurisdictions, they also cover a part of the accommodation, with the residents paying for the other portion. Often, the portion that the resident pays is called an accommodation fee, a co-payment, or a user fee, and in some jurisdictions, that fee may depend on the level of your income. Clarica Insurance notes that depending on the province you live in, your out-of-pocket expenses for facility care could be between $18,250 and $36,500 a year.

Tip

Long-term care insurance is discussed in Chapter 6, "Claiming Medical Expenses on Your Tax Return." This is coverage that can help with both home care and long-term facility care (nursing homes). While it is a fairly recent phenomenon in Canada, this type of insurance may be very worthwhile to help deal with some of the costs before you actually need care.

Insurance Canada reports that for certified facilities with government subsidies, typical long-term care facility costs can be as follows:

- A private room may cost $1901.23 per month.
- A semi-private room may cost $1597.06.
- A ward facility may cost $1353.73 (or $919.73 with an additional subsidy based on income).

There is a wide range of financial arrangements (cost sharing between the resident and the government), and these can differ from province to province, and even from health region to health region. Still, for seniors who require more living and health care support, a nursing home can be a very cost-effective choice if you qualify.

Medications are not usually covered in the nursing home (unlike in the hospital), and you will need to pay for these through your government-sponsored seniors' plan or any other plan you may have.

Facility Checklist

Here are some things to keep in mind when you are making choices about which facility you want to apply to:

- Usually, you are not guaranteed your first choice of facility. Ask about how the wait list works. For example, if you turn down an available room in one facility, do you lose your place in line?
- Once a room becomes available, you may be expected to accept it within 48 hours or lose it. Make sure you know what you want and also understand that there may be a period when you are paying for two accommodations: your current home or apartment and the new nursing home.
- Ask the administrator or the director for a full list of any extra charges, such as upgrades from double to single rooms.
- Ask for a list of the items that will be supplied by the facility and those you are responsible for buying

(cable, telephone, newspaper subscription, etc.). These differ from place to place.

- Find out what the facility will cover and what you will be responsible for covering with regard to special equipment like wheelchairs and walkers.
- Check the terms of away passes. If you take a trip away, you will still need to pay your portion of the fee; however, you will need to check whether the government will continue to pay its portion in your absence and for how long.
- Find out in advance who to contact, what recourse you have, and what higher authority you can go to if you want to register a complaint or if you suspect abuse.

Assistive Devices

Assistive devices are medical equipment, gadgets, and other aids and technologies that assist people in their daily activities. While they can be helpful for people of any age who are challenged in some way, seniors tend to be the most frequent users of assistive devices for things such as loss of balance, difficulty moving around, or hearing loss (for instance, over half of seniors experience some form of hearing loss). Today there are many devices that can help overcome these challenges.

The Public Health Agency of Canada presents the following chart on its website:

Task	Assistive Devices
Bathing	Grab bars, hand-held shower head, bath seat with arm rails, non-slip floor mat.
Dressing	Long-handled shoe horn, Velcro fastenings, sock pullers, rubber gloves (for gripping tight-fitting stockings).
Preparing food	Easy-grip utensils, side-opening oven door, height-adjustable cupboards and counters, automatic-stop kettle, pouring aid.
Eating	Easy-grip utensils, specially designed dishes.
Moving/physical activities	Cane, walker, wheelchair, slip-resistant flooring.
Using the telephone	Loud-ringing phone, flashing-light ring indicator, large numbers and buttons, automatic dialing, voice enhancement.
Doing the laundry	Main-floor laundry room, easy-access equipment.
Enjoying hobbies	Playing card holder, long-handled gardening tools, television remote control with large buttons and a captioning button.
Computers	Specialty computer stores carry items like screen-reading software that includes enlargement features for individuals with reduced vision. Voice recognition systems and modified keyboards and mice are also available for people with mobility and dexterity limitations.
Entering the home	Loud doorbell or flashing-light signal.
Securing your home	Automatic light device, personal or home alarm system, cell phone, thermostat control.

Source: *Assistive Devices Info Sheet for Seniors*, pages 2–3, www.phac-aspc.gc.ca/seniors-aines/pubs/info_sheets/assistive/index.htm, Public Health Agency of Canada, 2006. Reproduced with the permission of the Minister of Public Works and Government Services, 2006.

Half the battle in procuring an assistive device is knowing what you need and seeing if there is a device that is helpful. This may seem rather obvious, but we have come across many individuals who are utterly unaware that there are assistive devices to help their particular problem. We all know, for instance, about a cane or a walker for those with difficulty getting about. But did you know that there are devices that can help you put on socks or button your buttons? Nowadays there have been so many advancements in this area that it is wise for you to check with a number of sources to determine what is out there. Here is a partial list of sources that can help:

- Your doctor or nurse
- Your occupational therapist
- Brochures in health centres
- Magazines for seniors
- Pharmacies (Shoppers Drug Mart has an entire chain dedicated to providing home health care devices that can be either rented or purchased)
- Medical supply stores
- Associations for different conditions
- Hardware stores (for items like intercoms and special kitchen utensils with better grips)

Prescriptions and Assistive Devices

Some assistive devices, such as eyeglasses or hearing aids, need a prescription. These devices require an expert's assessment. Others are available over the counter. But even when they are available to you directly, it is good to consult an expert (a doctor, a nurse, an occupational therapist) so that you are fitted properly. For example, canes (somewhat as with hockey sticks) need to be the right height and able to support your weight. Some devices (such as braces for back problems) may need a professional in a specialty store to help fit them.

Coverage for Assistive Devices

Before running out and getting a device, you need to know who will pay for that item and what you will need to do to ensure that you get reimbursement.

Tip

As mentioned in Chapter 5, "Navigating Your Benefits Plans," and Chapter 6, "Claiming Medical Expenses on Your Tax Return," it is very important, especially for the more expensive devices, that you seek the help of a physician or other professional who is designated to assess your condition and prescribe a device. This will help you qualify for a complete or partial reimbursement from a funding or insurance agency. It will also be essential should you need to claim the expense on your income taxes.

Remember that even if you don't need a prescription to buy or rent the device, you should get your practitioner to write you one anyway. This will prove that it has been ordered by a qualified practitioner and may make the difference between getting reimbursement and not getting it.

GOVERNMENT PROGRAMS

It's always a good idea to start with the government to find out what program is available to you. The Resource Guide at the end of this chapter contains information about provincial and territorial contacts for assistive devices. Some provinces and territories have programs to help seniors or people with disabilities purchase the assistive devices they need at affordable prices or help with obtaining a bank loan. Once again, each jurisdiction has its own rules, and it is best to contact them directly. The important thing is to get in touch with them.

PRIVATE INSURANCE

If you are a senior who has some private insurance, find out what is covered, what you need, and how to claim.

COMMUNITY ORGANIZATIONS

Organizations such as Kiwanis, the Rotary Club, the Lions Club, or the Royal Canadian Legion may offer advice or assistance for procuring assistive devices.

Veterans Affairs Canada (VAC) offers a wide variety of programs and services to veterans and other eligible clients. Its health care program, Aids for Daily Living, assists clients with the purchase of assistive devices such as prosthetic and orthotic devices, walkers, canes, wheelchairs, etc. To learn more about the programs, services, and funding offered by VAC, contact your regional office (see the blue pages of your telephone directory under Government of Canada). If you have access to the

Internet, you can visit the VAC website at www.vac-acc.gc.ca.

There is a great deal of confusion over what the government provides and pays for, and what extended health care benefits cover you as a senior. This is in part a result of the fact that in Canada very little beyond hospitals and physicians is actually uniform. We mentioned in another chapter that "universal" health care doesn't mean "uniform" health care. You will need to understand exactly what benefits you are entitled to, and whether those benefits are for medication, home care, or supportive housing. When you are a senior, so much depends on your own personal situation and how you rate on the needs assessment. However, finding the information will be rewarding because often there are more supports in the system than people think.

Tip

If you are a senior, enlist help from your children, your friends, and your grandchildren to help you procure information on websites. The grandkids will love the challenge—they'll do almost anything to be legitimately glued to the screen of a computer.

Use the information in this chapter to guide them to the websites and organizations from which you need information so they don't come back with printed advice from snake-oil salesmen. But whatever you do, do not feel ashamed that you are having trouble figuring it all out. It is a very complex area. Why do we say this? Simple. This chapter was the most challenging of all to write.

Seniors frequently do not tap one resource: family and friends. Perhaps it is pride and a feeling of needing to be self-sufficient that stops a senior from asking for help. Perhaps it is a feeling that he or she is disturbing someone. Whether you are a senior or someone helping a senior, don't forget that you have a right to this information and to assistance help. Dig to get the answers you need.

RESOURCE GUIDE

BOOKS, GUIDES, AND MAGAZINES

The Complete Aging and Caregiving Resource Guide
www.caregiver.on.ca
This website was developed from June Callwood's television show *Caregiving with June Callwood.* It is a great resource for anyone taking care of a parent, a spouse, or themselves, and it provides a fairly complete list of federal and provincial resources and services that are available. It can be downloaded free of charge, but you will need Adobe Acrobat to read it.

Parenting Your Parents: Support Strategies for Meeting the Challenges of Aging in the Family. Bart J. Mindszenthy and Michael Gordon (Toronto: Dundurn Press, 2005).

This book uses case studies and gives advice on how to manage the aging process of a loved one. It has an incredible resource guide.

Comfort Life Magazine
www.comfortlife.ca
Telephone: (905) 272-1843
This magazine is dedicated to retirement living and health care options in Canada. This is a terrific magazine for anyone seeking information on options. It has great articles and resource guides.

GOVERNMENT PROGRAMS

Government of Canada
www.seniors.gc.ca
Seniors Canada On-Line is a wonderful website that will help you access all kinds of resources that are available to you by province or territory. It will link you up with government offices, agencies, associations, books and guides, and other resources in your jurisdiction and across Canada. This website is the easiest way to get links to your province's centre for information and other resources all at the same time.

To navigate the website, click on the area of the home page that interests you. For example, if you are interested in funded nursing home options, click on "Housing." The next page will give you a list of the types of housing available. You would click on "Retirement homes." The next page will provide you with a map of Canada, where you can click on the right jurisdiction. Should you return to the same website, it will usually recall the jurisdiction that was last requested, so if you want to look for information on another you will need to click "Change your location" on the left, under "Tools."

The Public Health Agency of Canada
www.phac-aspc.gc.ca
The Public Health Agency of Canada offers a wonderful summary of assistive devices and a linked guide to all the provincial and territorial websites where you can find information.

To navigate the site, click on the bar marked "Seniors," then scroll down to "Seniors Issues" and click on "Assistive Devices—Info Sheet for Seniors" or "Go For It!" See also Chapter 2: Steps Involved.

Home Adaptations
www.canadabenefits.gc.ca
Under "I Am," choose "A Senior," then scroll down to Home Adaptations for Seniors Independence (HASI) or go directly to www.cmhc-schl.gc.ca/cmhc-schl/en/co/prfinas/prfinas_004.cfm.
Telephone: 1-800-668-2642
TTY: 1-613-748-2447

CANADIAN ON-LINE PHARMACIES

Of the many on-line pharmacies today, here is one that is based in Canada:
Canada Drugs.com
www.canadadrugs.com
Telephone: 1-800-796-6209

ELEVEN

Navigating End-of-Life Care

We hope readers won't be tempted to skip this chapter—we know that some people avoid having discussions about the end of life, and others feel there won't be anything relevant for them right now and can put it off. But thinking about the way our lives—and those of our loved ones—come to an end is not something to be ignored. By reading this chapter, you will arm yourself with the information you will need to deal with the health system when someone in your family needs end-of-life care. We're starting with Francesca's own story.

> At 7:30 P.M., on July 8, 2003, at our family home, my father, Dr. Roberto Grosso, died. Just two months earlier, I had given birth to a baby girl, Giulia. Because I was a new mother, my family spared me from being involved in many of the difficult,

emotional decisions that went into caring for my dad in the last months of his life. My father had been diagnosed with cancer only 18 months prior to his death and had undergone a very difficult operation that has a high mortality rate. As a family, we went through the rollercoaster of emotions: the horror at an unexpected diagnosis; the tension and fear waiting for the results of the assessment to decide whether he was a candidate for surgery; the relief when the CT scan revealed that the cancer seemed contained, and that he was indeed a candidate for surgery; the prayers we sent up during the operation, saying we would be grateful if he just pulled through.

He did survive the operation. We were filled with hope that somehow his death from this cancer was not meant to be. We hoped that the success of the operation was a sign that his time was not up. We became cautiously optimistic when the first test results came back that my father was "clean." And as the months passed and we approached the first big hurdle, which was, in his case, the one-year mark of cancer-free tests, this optimism grew.

But it was not to be.

I received the call where I worked, in the office of the Ontario minister of health. My father called himself. His voice was calm, almost clinical, yet defeated. His message was short and simple: "Francesca, I have cancer in my liver. I will live for three months. Your papa is dying. Do not get on the Internet and read all those things. There is nothing to be done in my case."

The routine liver test confirmed that the cancer had spread. Being a doctor himself, he knew the reality that not all cancers are created equal, and that his was a specifically sinister and lethal variety. My world exploded.

In the minister's office, I had helped deliver countless difficult cases into the hands of the great men and women of medicine; these were situations in which the hope of seeing a "top doctor" held the promise of cure. Yet once I had managed to get people into the "right" place for treatment, the case for me was closed. Who knew what happened after that? My job had been done, and I rejoiced in my small victories.

I never saw the path these people faced, probably because I didn't want to. Now I had come face to face with that long, difficult path when access to the best care the system offers doesn't fix the problem and you are left to navigate a health care system under the most stressed emotional conditions.

For the first time, I could not pick up the phone and solve the problem. The problem was that my father was dying, and there was no one to whom I could turn to stop it from happening.

We all know that death is part of life, but somehow we remain unprepared—possibly because we feel that allowing ourselves to prepare for death is somehow a denial of life. Certainly there are no shortages of emotional support and advice, from clinics, social workers, books, and Dr. Phil and his ilk. The two of us are not qualified to provide solutions for the psychological issues, but we will attempt to add some constructive direction to help make managing the process of caring for a dying loved one easier. In this chapter, we hope to provide some much-needed insight into how our health system works and what is available to you and your loved one in the way of supports. The Resource Guide at the end of the chapter will help you navigate your way to more information, documents, and services.

Understanding Palliative Care

Palliative care seems like such a straightforward concept, yet it is wrought with heart-tugging implications. Let's begin by explaining the difference between someone who is a palliative care candidate and someone who is terminal—because there is a difference. Palliative care is a philosophy of care that deals with the management of disturbing symptoms like pain. Palliative care is not the active treatment of the disease itself, which will ultimately lead to death. Let us take the example of a cancer patient who has maxed out on all treatments to cure or arrest the disease. That person could live for months or years, but there is no active treatment left that holds the promise of curing, stopping, or reversing the disease. That patient, once in palliative care, will not receive any further interventions of a curative nature.

Once a patient is assessed as a candidate for palliative care, the doctor—and it can be the family doctor, a specialist, or the hospital doctor—makes a referral to palliative care services. The referral is important because a palliative care patient is entitled to certain services, at home or in the community, that are covered by medicare in his or her province or territory. These services can include doctor visits at home (along with visits from other practitioners), services, and equipment. Also, a palliative care patient is eligible to be admitted into a palliative care facility if the home option is not the right one for the patient and his or her family or caregivers, and if there is a facility that has space.

Although a palliative care patient will receive no further active treatment for the disease that will lead ultimately to death, this does *not* mean that the patient will not be treated for other conditions or diseases that affect his or her comfort and quality of life. For example, if a patient develops an infection that is treatable with antibiotics, and if that infection causes discomfort, he or she will be treated.

Sometimes palliative care patients can get treatments, such as "palliative radiation," that would be used to treat a disease in non-palliative care patients. But in these cases, the treatments serve a different purpose. They are done to manage symptoms, largely to relieve pain, and not to cure or treat the disease itself. Take, for instance, a patient who has a tumour in his throat that causes him to choke. The tumour is not operable, is not treatable, and will spread throughout the body. Ultimately the patient will die. However, the doctor may order palliative radiation, which will reduce the size of the tumour. This will enhance the patient's comfort, and it may prolong life to the extent that it reduces or postpones the possibility of choking.

Today, the modern palliative care philosophy is to ensure that patients can live as long as they can in comfort.

Francesca recalls one woman asking, "Why do they call it 'palliative care treatment'? Where's the treatment?" The answer is that there is treatment, but it is different from the treatment you would get for a curable disease. Here's what you can expect from palliative care regardless of where you live in Canada:

- There will be no active treatments or interventions for the underlying disease.
- There will be active treatment for pain.
- If the patient is in a setting that offers palliative care services, he or she will not be taken to the hospital if something goes wrong. There will be no heart massages and other interventions. In short, no heroic measures will be taken to prevent death.

A friend of Francesca's was incensed to find out that her grandmother would no longer be eligible to have her hemoglobin levels tested once she was considered a palliative care patient. In her grandmother's case, those levels were tested to determine if treatment—a blood transfusion—was necessary. Once the patient was declared palliative, no more interventions would take place. Why do tests if you aren't going to do anything about the results?

This is not to say that no tests will be done at all. It may still be in order to monitor things like INR (international normalized ratio) levels in your blood, which measure the anti-coagulant effect of blood-thinning medication. Tests that help measure medication doses so that the patient is comfortable and not being overdosed would also still be done. But those tests that are normally done to decide on an active treatment would be stopped.

What you can expect from palliative care is good pain management and the management of other symptoms of the process of dying so that your loved one dies in as much comfort as possible. That is what palliative care treatment is about.

Understanding Terminal Care

"Terminal" refers to the final stages of life, when the patient's death is imminent. Here we can see the trajectory of death very clearly. As in palliative care, the focus is on managing the patient's symptoms to provide comfort. But in this stage, the management of symptoms is very intense. The patient may lose consciousness as a result of the illness. The medication doses to manage pain may be high enough at this stage to contribute to coma or even slightly premature death. But the alternative would be an agonizing existence for the patient. In this stage, other peripheral diseases, like infections, will not be treated. The discomfort they may cause is the sole focus of treatment.

It is important to be aware that intense symptom management at this terminal stage may in fact lead to premature death, as we suggested above. The intent is not to end the patient's life but rather to provide for the adequate amount of pain management, which in turn may have a hand in a slightly premature death.

These concepts are very important. Take, for instance, the woman who is very pleased with her gynecologist until she wants to terminate her pregnancy and then discovers that her doctor, based on religious beliefs, will not assist her in this process. It is essential that you discuss the "world views" of the person providing care to make certain they are consistent with your own. It is very important that your care provider understand and accommodate your expectations of palliative and terminal care, in particular with regard to the following:

- your religious and personal beliefs and preferences;
- the doctor's willingness to actively treat conditions other than the underlying disease (you may or may not want to go to someone who would not treat, for instance, a urinary tract infection and will only provide pain management);
- the doctor's views on providing intense management of pain, even if it might prematurely end your loved one's life.

This final question is very important. There is no right or wrong answer, and it really depends on the beliefs of the patient and his or her loved ones.

Dr. Michael Gordon, a leading geriatrician who has a strong interest in medical ethics, says that many religions are not opposed to rigorous pain management at the very last stage of life. This applies even if the pain management may prematurely end life by a few hours (because the intent is not to end the patient's life but to make him or her comfortable). We understand that in Judaism and Catholicism, the relief of suffering is very important, and that the focus of care should be directed to symptom management with whatever treatments are available. Still, Dr. Gordon explains that some religions may address the issue differently. So you need to know not only how you and your loved ones feel about it, but also how the doctor feels about it. You all need to be on the same page.

Make certain that your doctor doesn't have the philosophy of over-medicating when it isn't necessary. Most good doctors won't, but it doesn't hurt to ask your family doctor to refer you to a specialist who has a good reputation for palliative care and doesn't over-medicate. Most doctors who have been trained in palliative care, and whose training is updated, will not over-medicate. If your own family doctor provides the care, make it clear that it is very important to your loved one and to you that he or she not be over-medicated. Sometimes raising it as an issue is enough to make your doctor mindful of your concerns, which may impact his or her decisions on pain medication. The whole idea of palliative care is that palliative patients should live as long as they can in comfort. Intense medication is part of the final stage of pain management. But you will want to ensure, before your loved one is terminal, that your doctor is allowing him or her to experience as good a quality of life as possible.

Usually in these situations, the patient and his or her loved ones are divided in their ability to accept the implications of the palliative care assessment. Usually, the loved one accepts the assessment until the actual treatment plans are being made. Then she fights the treatment plans because she really hasn't accepted the diagnosis. Thus a loved one, without intending to do so, can become a barrier to providing the patient with the comfort and support needed. She remains stuck on trying to ensure active treatment in the hopes of changing the diagnosis. This often leads to a disconnect in the decision-making process on how to proceed with care; even if loved ones who are in denial are not the personal care attorney, they can put sufficient pressure on the others. It is not, as we said earlier, within the scope of this chapter, or within the realm of our knowledge, to provide psychological methods to deal with this issue. However, recognizing someone's failure to accept the palliative diagnosis and its implications is key to managing the situation effectively. If you see it happening, you would be well advised to seek professional help (your caregiver can direct you to the appropriate services) because this type of denial can really affect the quality of the last few months or weeks of a person's life.

Francesca saw first-hand with her father that all his medical needs were taken care of by the system. The emotional needs are something quite separate, however, and very often patients' families have trouble distinguishing between the two. This may seem like a self-evident point. It isn't. Often people think that because their loved one is dying, he or she should be entitled to around-the-clock care—that a nurse or someone should be there to help attend to the patient if he or she wants something. Sometimes family members believe that a dying person should not be left alone.

All these needs are quite important. Francesca recalls, "Despite his rational, clinical training as a surgeon, my father was afraid to die. I have never seen anyone die with more dignity, but my father had times when he was afraid to be alone, afraid of what death would feel like, and afraid most of all of the process of death. He needed support. He needed people sitting near him. He needed to hold our hands. He needed his pillows constantly adjusted and his leg constantly moved. He had very important and very visceral needs."

But these are not medical needs. In Canada, our medicare system is designed to deal largely with medical needs, not social or emotional support. Though we can expect some free counselling from staff social workers at hospitals or other institutions, the heavy lifting on the emotional front is left to our loved ones. It is the family or close friends who must provide those supports—either by doing it themselves or by hiring someone to sit with the patient when they cannot be there.

Acute Care Services in Hospitals

Some acute care hospitals are affiliated with a palliative care services centre or offer their own palliative care services within the hospital. An acute care hospital is not the place to send a loved one who is a palliative care patient and is not in need of acute care services. Acute care is not for someone who is very ill; it is for patients who need intervention to treat an urgent problem. People who are palliative may need acute care to treat a secondary problem like an infection, but the underlying condition will not be cured by intervention. Many people get confused on this point. Take, for instance, a very ill person who is admitted to the hospital with her lungs filling with fluid. Her lungs are drained, but the hospital finds that her heart is weakening, she is inoperable, and she will not recover from the heart problem. There is no treatment that will stop the heart's deterioration. She is declared a palliative care patient and the hospital wants her out.

One can only imagine the reaction of the family. How can a hospital turn away a patient who is so obviously ill? Isn't the hospital exactly the place for cases like this? This situation is very common, as is the reaction.

To understand the hospital's position and deal with it effectively rather than waging war, you must learn what acute care hospitals do and don't do. Every week we can pick up the paper and read about overcrowding in our hospitals. While we often blame governments and institutions for this reality, each of us must accept a certain amount of responsibility for using the hospital inappropriately when we should be putting our efforts into finding the right setting for our needs or the needs of our loved ones. Hospital doctors will inform you when they conclude that the hospital is no longer the place for your loved one. We are not suggesting that governments have done everything right and that there are no problems to solve. We know there are issues that governments still need to deal with. As Michael pointed out in his book *Four Strong Winds*, the hospital used to be the hub for everything. Today it is not.

We now realize that the hospital is the most expensive venue in which to treat patients. The acute care hospital has to deal with patients who may need urgent surgery or who go into cardiac arrest and need intervention. Hospitals have to have the right number of staff on site at all times to deal with scheduled and unscheduled procedures and events that require emergency or complex care. These people are trained to deal with acute care. The building itself has to contain all the state-of-the-art equipment to deal with the most urgent situations. That's why the cost of delivering care in an acute care hospital is so high. The average cost of a one-day stay in hospital for the average patient, not including surgery or any other intervention, is about $1000. To be effective, hospitals need beds for those who require some kind of intervention and who can benefit from acute care. Palliative care patients need a place where their disturbing symptoms will be treated and they will be made comfortable—full stop. That is not an acute care hospital.

Tip

Understand what needs the system will and will not cover so you can better plan your support system.

Palliative Care Settings

With an understanding of the difference between emotional and medical needs and between palliative and terminal care, you will be better able to make choices about where the patient should be cared for. Palliative care is becoming more widely available in a host of different community settings, including the following:

- Hospitals that have wings that provide palliative care treatment
- Complex continuing care settings that house patients with many complex conditions and chronic diseases
- Long-term care settings (nursing homes, retirement homes)
- Free-standing hospices
- Home care settings

Not long ago, few nursing homes offered palliative care services. There was even a time when intravenous tubes and feeding tubes were not allowed in nursing homes. But there has been a massive shift in the type of care nursing homes can deliver. Today some of these institutions provide palliative care and some do not.

Governments are also beginning to demand that complex continuing care services be offered in a variety of community settings. Given that a person can receive palliative care at home, it would stand to reason that he or she should be able to get this type of care in other community settings as well..

In Ontario and other jurisdictions, palliative care is becoming part of the mandate of nursing homes. But as with other areas of health care, services across Canada are not uniform. Jurisdictions make changes at different stages from one another. Here are some things you should find out about various settings or programs you may be considering:

- What palliative care support does the facility or program offer?
- If it is a setting with an in-house doctor, what is that doctor's philosophy?
- Does the program have volunteers? This is important since programs with volunteers tend to be more wide-ranging in the types of supports they provide.

When a nursing home does *not* provide palliative care, it is more a place of residence for the elderly with supportive living programs, meals, and entertainment. It will probably have some medical monitoring when there is a problem with residents who need medical attention. In these types of nursing homes, doctors do rounds to check if residents are in need of medical attention, and they instruct the nursing home to call an ambulance if there is a problem.

Unlike an acute care hospital, an institution that provides palliative care services has a staff trained to deal with keeping a patient comfortable during the last stages of life. Although there are nurses and doctors and social workers, the doctors' functions are very different from those in an acute care hospital. These doctors will assess patients and medications and treatments for the sole purpose of making the patient comfortable.

Francesca has seen many people who are admitted to hospital and feel relieved to be there for a while, even after having been declared palliative. Maybe it's because they are in denial, or maybe it's because it is comforting to think that if something were to go wrong, the hospital staff would be able to somehow thwart imminent danger. She has also noted, however, that as time progressed and these patients saw that they were not going to get better, they started missing home, their bed, their things.

Home Care and Making the Care Decision

Let's continue with Francesca's story. "My father wanted to die at home, perhaps because he saw the reality of the institutional setting. My father wanted to enjoy being upstairs and hearing us coming, going, and eating together, even if he couldn't be at the table. Of course, he also wanted to feel comfortable, and he would be more comfortable at home. We gave him a bell to ring and later we realized that a baby monitor was an excellent tool to use to hear him if he needed anything. But he made us promise that no matter how difficult it got, we wouldn't put him into an institution. And he was a doctor! So I figure that if he didn't want to go anywhere but home, it's a pretty good argument for better care at home. I need to remind myself and anyone in this situation that frequently, while we are allowing ourselves to be immersed in the logistics of medical care, we might stop appreciating, even if for a moment, that a human life needs meaning. For my dad, home was meaning."

There is evidence that suggests that patients who go home actually live a little longer. Ninety percent of all Canadians want to die at home, yet the sad truth is that fewer than 50 percent have the support that allows them to do that. But such a statistic doesn't address the reasons behind the relatively small number of people who actually do die at home, much less provide solutions to possible challenges.

The fact is that for many families, bringing a patient home isn't easy. And if something were to go terribly wrong, caregivers are afraid they would not know what to do. We probably tend to ask ourselves: Wouldn't the patient be better off in a facility? Many people panic when a loved one who is at the end of life shows signs of dying. Their breath might become more laboured. The first thing many people want to do is call 911. Actually that is the last thing to do. When you call 911, your loved one will end up in an acute care hospital, which, as explained above, is usually not the place for them.

Francesca recalls, "The concern we had with my father was less about emergency in the sense of calling a doctor. It had to do with what we would do if something were to go wrong all of a sudden and we were left not knowing how to make my father comfortable. What would we do? Supposed he had trouble breathing? Put rather simply and perhaps crudely, how do we deal with the more unpleasant symptoms of the process of death?"

When a family has to confront what to do with a palliative care patient, it is important to consider the needs of the patient. However, it is also very important that you ask yourself two fundamental questions: How much emotional support will my loved one get at home, and are we, the family, able to handle the death process emotionally? Many families and patients feel safer and less vulnerable when they know there are people always around. Also, there are certain situations where you do need your loved one to be in an institution. For example, when a patient is still mobile but prone to falling, it can sometimes be impossible for the family caregiver to lift him or her up. Some people have depended on the fire department to come and help. If this becomes a frequent occurrence, it may be best to have the person in an institution.

Francesca understands some of the concerns family members have in deciding between a palliative care facility and home care. She lists the common ones below and then offers a number of practical tips to deal with some of these concerns. She has tried to separate the medical concerns from the practical concerns and the emotional ones. Frequently, the list of concerns seems insurmountable. At the end of the chapter, in the Resource Guide, you will find contact organizations, numbers, and websites to help you navigate as you weigh your options.

1. No one can stay home 24 hours a day with my loved one.
2. Even if someone could, we don't want to because we're scared. We're scared to take care of our loved one because we aren't doctors or nurses, and we don't know what to do if something goes wrong.
3. My loved one can't get up from bed alone or bathe and feed herself. In a facility they do these things. We are afraid to do that at home.
4. Our loved one needs specialized equipment like a hospital bed that can be raised and lowered.
5. My loved one needs specific tests or medications like morphine that must be delivered intravenously at specific intervals. How do we do that? What if one of us falls asleep when the medication needs to be administered into the intravenous system?
6. What do I do when my loved one dies?

How Home Care Works

To begin to answer these questions, it is important to compare the services the patient would get in a palliative care clinic to what can be provided at home. As discussed above, in a facility medical needs would be completely taken care of. Medications and pain management would be monitored. But someone would *not* be sitting by the patient's bed 24 hours a day. The patient would be alone in his or her room much of the time. The staff would check in on the patient, but it would still be up to the family, friends, and/or help hired by the family to provide that additional level of support and comfort. So the onus of providing emotional support would fall on the family in both settings.

At home, a patient's medical needs would be taken care of by home-care services. Visits by a home care professional and other services are covered by your provincial health insurance depending on the province you live in. At the moment, provincial governments have promised a certain set of services for palliative care patients. You may have heard this referred to as a "basket of services." Most provinces and regions have these supports in place, and for the most part they offer terrific service covered by medicare. But you always need to ask exactly what is covered and for how long. Some things are covered for a finite number of weeks or months. The coordinator for the patient's care can usually answer these questions, so there is no need to call someone at your provincial government.

How do you get the services of these home care personnel—doctors, nurses, and others? If their services are covered by medicare, the doctor or care provider needs to order them. The home care team coördinates care. Your care provider (often the doctor) needs to *fill out the home care application* when you have made your decision and conveyed it to him or her. This doctor can be someone in an acute care hospital, your family physician, or a specialist. In the hospital, the doctor signs the application, and all arrangements are made through the hospital discharge planner with the community home care agency. You do not need to make these arrangements yourself. Medications, tests, and necessary devices would be included in the instructions given to the home care agency. You may need to pay a small rental fee on some devices, but usually the charges are all covered for a certain number of months if they have been ordered by the doctor and if the patient is in the hospital, dispatched by the discharge planner. For example, your loved one may need morphine to be delivered intravenously. It will be delivered by people trained to install, set up, and monitor the "cad pump"—the device used to deliver the drug automatically at the right time—and these same people will replace the pump with new cartridges when needed.

Once the patient is discharged from hospital, the home care agency takes over and further assesses the patient's needs. There are two important people you want to have a good relationship with: the discharge planner in the hospital and the contact for the home care people. Often the hospital will have a social worker help provide support to the family, and he or she can report back to the discharge planner if something more needs to be considered for proper care. But if you establish a bond with them, these are the people who can help you with things like accessing better rental equipment. For example, there is the standard walker device and then there's the upgraded model with a hand brake and a place where the patient can sit. You'd rather have the one with the features that will help the patient, wouldn't you? It is a matter of human nature—people who are treated with kindness tend to respond in kind. Establishing good relationships with key decision-makers is as important in health care as it is anywhere else. If you've made an ally out of the person who will plan your loved one's care, there is often some room for her to spring for a few bells and whistles—if she can.

Tip

Discharge planners in hospitals and case managers in community health agencies are tired, busy, and always dealing with stressed families who often read them the riot act. A nice disposition and kindness on your part can go a long way.

In the case of Francesca's father, members of his care team came a few times a day. (Of course, the frequency will depend on the level of care needed.) They monitored how much medication he was getting and reported back to the doctor or somebody who would update the course of treatment if needed. These workers also bathed him in bed and dressed his bedsores, which were more of a problem toward the end of his life. They kept detailed charts that the next person coming could consult to continue the care. A doctor came by as well, sometimes every day.

Francesca's family didn't hire extra help because there was always someone at home. They left the medical care to the home care workers, and the family spent their time talking to her father and doing things like holding his hand and moving his pillows. For them, it was more important to provide the emotional support at home.

Make sure you don't leave the hospital without understanding the plan that has been put in place for your loved one, and make sure that you have the name and contact number of the community home care coordinator assigned to your case. This is key. It's a good idea to have the name and number of the discharge planner of the hospital, too. The home care coordinator will be in charge of scheduling who will come to your house, making sure your rentals are ordered, and dealing with any issues that arise with home care. Ask him what services will be covered. These can range from personal care to physiotherapy for the purpose of relieving uncomfortable symptoms. But if it is something like physiotherapy, it will have to be ordered through the doctor. In short, "Grandma would like some physiotherapy" won't cut it. If you see a need, on the other hand, be sure to talk to the coordinator about it. He will conduct an assessment, and if he finds that extra treatment is needed, he will start the ball rolling in getting it ordered.

Tip

A person is eligible for supports such as physiotherapy without having been in the hospital, but the services must be ordered through your doctor, who will fill out the referral for home care, indicating that the patient is to receive palliative care. You will get a call from home care to arrange the visits. Once home care is established, the same routes are followed for accessing extra treatments or helpful devices.

Though it's rare, a patient may be entitled to have medicare pay for someone to do some house cleaning and grocery shopping. This entitlement depends on the program available in his or her province, territory, or region. For example, if a patient lived with an elderly husband who was limited in what he could do, these services might be ordered and covered under medicare. This would be in addition to the professionals coming to the house to manage her care. A doctor would visit her if required. She could have things like a hospital bed or other equipment ordered through home care if the doctor thought it necessary.

Someone should be at home with the patient at all times. But many people are afraid to be left alone with someone who is dying in case his or her condition worsens. Breathing problems are particularly common among people who are bedridden for a long time. Ask your home care worker if oxygen can be brought if the patient's breathing will become laboured. Home care will bring oxygen and show you how it works—it is easy. But it is important to have two people present when new equipment is brought in so they can both be trained. They can then show the others what to do. In palliative care, there is often not a lot to do except spend time with the patient, but you will certainly want more than one person to know simple things like how to turn on the oxygen.

In Francesca's father's case, and to illustrate the sophistication of home care devices, two units of oxygen were brought in. One operated with electricity and one didn't, in case of a power outage. Francesca remembers being very impressed with that level of detail.

Today, home care equipment is well designed and simple to use. And most of this equipment has been designed so it can be brought into the home. Gone are the days when you couldn't get a hospital bed except in the hospital. Almost everything is now available for home use, and will be brought and set up for you if it is considered necessary. If the device is simple, the family can set it up themselves. For more complex devices, home-care services will coordinate the set-up.

Hiring Extra Help

There may be other reasons to consider hiring someone beyond what is medically necessary and provided by home care. Many people are comfortable only if there are trained personnel at their side caring for their loved one. If you are the sole family member looking after the patient when home care workers aren't there, you need to be sure you get a good night's sleep but you don't want to leave the patient alone. You might decide to hire someone to sit with the patient at night. You might also need help during the day so you can go out or attend to matters no one else can look after. If the patient is in a palliative care facility, you might hire a personal duty nurse or a personal care worker to provide comfort, company, and support to the patient when you can't be there.

A nurse obviously has training that a personal care worker doesn't have. A nurse can provide a certain level of clinical care. A personal care worker is someone who can provide support. She can do all kinds of domestic things, like prepare meals, bathe the person, provide housekeeping support, and help move your loved one. Mostly she can provide you with the peace of mind that comes from knowing that someone else is there at all times, and that you can go to sleep and someone will be keeping the bedside vigil. You have to know what you feel you need—you may feel better with a nurse around, but medically there may not be a need—and what you can afford.

Case coordinators in home care agencies will help locate trained people through organizations that provide nurses and other supports on a rotating basis. If your loved one is in the hospital, the discharge planner can help direct you to agencies that provide these services. The hospital will not hire this person on your behalf, but it will give you lists of agencies. Get the names of several agencies with full contact information. Ask the doctor or the discharge planner at the hospital if he or she feels your loved one needs around-the-clock *nursing* care. Often palliative care patients do not need such intensive care. Usually you need a good personal care worker. A nurse is both more expensive and often unnecessary, since nurses will be coming to provide specialized care.

Tip

Be very, very candid with the home care coordinator about the home situation so that he or she can order the most appropriate services.

With a palliative care patient another difficult truth to come to terms with is that something will inevitably go wrong. The process of death can be frightening. Someone like a nurse might provide the level of comfort you need to make you feel less afraid about dealing with the death process. He or she can also help you emotionally just by being there as the condition worsens. A nurse or personal care worker can be hired to be there for as many hours as is needed. But this will need to be paid out of your own pocket.

When the End Comes

The last concern, which is terrifying for most, surrounds what to do when your loved one dies. This is a question that is usually answered well by the doctor and the funeral home representative or director. They will tell you exactly what to do. Near the final stages of the patient's life, the family is wise to begin to make arrangements with a funeral home. Typically upon your loved one's death, you will make two phone calls. The first is to the doctor (or to the person or organization your doctor advises you to call). A doctor will come to pronounce your loved one dead and sign the death certificate. Your second call is to the funeral home. They will arrive to remove the body. If they arrive sooner, they will simply wait until the doctor has completed the necessary steps to declare the person dead. The funeral home will remove the body, but be aware that this can be a very traumatic experience, since the body is often placed in a body bag.

Financial Supports in the System

It is important to check what home care services are covered under medicare. Each province differs slightly in what it provides, and of course it also depends on the specifics of the case. If your grandmother doesn't live alone, she may not be entitled to housekeeping or grocery services, and if you want those services for her, you will have to pay for them yourself. But if she does live alone, or with someone who is not capable of doing these things, they may be provided and covered by medicare.

If you think you need private help, either at home or at a palliative care facility, the issue of cost is bound to factor in to your decision. Additional supports for the emotional needs of the patient or family are not covered through home care or at a palliative care facility. The average registered nurse costs about $36 to $40 per hour. However, it's likely that for a palliative care patient, an RN is not needed for supplementary help and emotional support, and certainly not 24 hours a day. A personal care worker would usually be fine. Agencies provide these services, as discussed, and a personal care worker is a great deal less expensive.

Having someone sit by Grandma's side and give her one-to-one care around the clock is comforting. Understand that you'll need to pay for this extra help—whether at home or in a palliative care facility.

There is also another support in the system that is new. The federal government has created a program called "Compassionate Care Leave Benefit" that allows eligible employees up to six weeks of paid benefits to care for a seriously ill or dying family member. This would be similar to maternity leave. During the time you're away, your employer cannot fire you. Your job is protected by laws passed by the government. The difference between this insurance and maternity leave insurance is that it can be split up and claimed by a few people—so you could take a couple of weeks and a sister or brother could take a couple of weeks. There is an inaugural waiting period of two weeks, during which no benefits will be paid; this is followed by a maximum of six weeks of leave. (So you get paid for six weeks but can be off for eight.) The benefit pays out 55 percent of your earnings, to a maximum payout of $413 per week. Each caregiver can make a claim so long as the total number of weeks claimed does not exceed eight. The Resource Guide at the end of this chapter provides the address for the Health Council of Canada website, where you can download an extensive report created to explain this benefit. You'll also find the website address for Human Resources and Social Development Canada, where you can download the forms you will need to apply.

Another significant cost is medication. As Michael notes in Chapter 13, "Navigating Canadian Health Care—Safely," since 1997 the second spending category after hospitals was drugs. In the hospital, medications are covered, but once you're outside the financially protective walls of the hospital, the picture changes. Unfortunately, medication coverage is one area in home care where there is a great deal of discrepancy. Rules differ according to provinces. In most provinces, not all drugs are covered in the home care setting. Your doctor or home care coordinator should be able to tell you whether the medications prescribed are covered in your province. Often, medications delivered directly into the body by special devices that are brought by home care workers are covered by the service. In addition, seniors in most provinces have a drug plan sponsored by the province, making continued drug therapy outside a hospital a much more affordable proposition. However, it is important to note that palliative home care is not only for the elderly. Younger people who are without drug plans are also palliative care patients, so it is important to check exactly what your province covers outside the hospital, whether in the home or in the palliative care facility.

Managing the Medications

Managing medications is a recurring theme of this book. In this discussion, the concern has less to do with adverse drug effects than it does with potential drug interactions. Typically in home care and palliative care, a doctor and a care coordinator are managing the situation. They should know every medication the patient is taking—usually they will have been ordered through them. When the patient is taking medications or supplements outside of the prescriptions ordered by the coordinating palliative care doctor, it is good to let them know.

The bigger concern here is dosages being administered by different family members. It is helpful to keep a log beside the bed so that if there are questions, you know who administered the last dose. While cure or improvement in condition is not the goal of palliative care, the patient's comfort is. And most of the medications are geared to that end. Administering too much or too little undermines the entire philosophy of the treatment. Above all, do not rely on the patient to remember when he or she got the last dose.

Your Own Personal Care Wishes

Once you go through the experience of attending the death of a loved one, certain things become apparent. One of these is the importance of sorting out your own choices in advance—basic planning. Francesca comes from a close family, but she was not prepared for the tension-induced bickering that cropped up over issues that today don't seem so important. If there were already major issues or tensions in the family, these would surely have reached a fever pitch during the tense and emotional time of her father's death. All unpleasant family problems tend to rise to the surface at times like this. Fights between family members have a good chance of graduating into all-out wars.

You can lessen the potential for conflict in your own end-of-life care by dealing upfront with the difficult legal decisions and providing advance directives to your loved ones so they will know how you want to be treated at the end of your life.

Advance directives outline your personal wishes for end-of-life care. These decisions, when not made by you in advance, are often the cause of tensions and fights among those caring for you. We may define death as the moment when we take our last breath, but our ability to make decisions for ourselves may be gone well before that, which is why these directives must be taken in advance of being ill—in short, when you are well.

There are two things you need in writing. The first is a Power of Attorney for Personal Care. This is a document that entrusts another person with the decision-making power in the event of your inability to make your own health care decisions. The document refers to the Substitute Decisions Act, which is basically the law that governs the point at which a person is considered to have become unable to make his or her own decisions. This is important because you don't want decisions being made by your attorney for personal care when you could be making them despite your illness. The act protects you on this point, so you don't need to worry about defining when you would hand over the decision-making authority to someone else. You should also choose an alternative attorney in case something happens to the first person you named.

The second thing you need to sign, which is typically part of the same power of attorney, is a document that outlines any special instructions you wish to have carried out on your behalf if you are incapable of making such a decision. Typically, this would be a clause stating something like this:

> I do not wish to have my life unduly prolonged by any course of treatment or any other medical procedure which offers no reasonable expectation of my recovering from life-threatening physical or mental incapacity, except as may be necessary for the relief of suffering.

This is a fairly standard clause and basically means that you agree to no heroic measures if you are very close to death and there isn't any reasonable expectation that you will recover—if that is what you want. Such a declaration will spare your loved ones a great deal of agony, especially if they are confronted with signing a DNR

(Do Not Resuscitate) order. Usually the family is asked to sign such an order when the patient is considered palliative.

Lawyers will typically include this language and will not necessarily discuss with you other decisions or options, but there are others. The list of websites and books we provide at the end of the chapter will help you consider your advance directives more fully.

As important as signing a DNR is, it is not the only important, tough decision your loved ones will need to make for which you could provide some advance direction. Certainly it is difficult to plan for all possible events, but there is something else you should specify—that is, where do you want to die if there are no more treatments available to you?

Francesca's family was lucky in that her father had always, since she was a child, told them that he wanted to die in his own bed. Having seen a number of friends and family go through similar events, she has come to believe that this is not the norm. In a typical situation, no one really knows where the patient would prefer to live out his or her last days and the family is confronted with having to ask this of the patient at the most difficult time. Sometimes they have agonizing battles with other family members or close friends over this point. Even if everyone has your best interests at heart, they will have different opinions that may reflect their personal preferences or fears, rather than your own. Taking care of a loved one at home when you don't know what to expect can be frightening, as we've said. Many find comfort in an institution that is staffed with people who are trained and "know what to do." In trying to do right by you, loved ones will still have different views. If you feel strongly one way or the other, make it clear. Put it in writing and talk to your family and your attorney for personal care.

What age is best to get these legal issues or personal preferences organized? None of us knows exactly when we are going to die or the circumstances, so there is no time like the present.

Tip

You don't need a lawyer to prepare the documents we've discussed so long as you have them witnessed.

A Note to Caregivers

Whether your loved one is in an institution or is having home care, the following points apply to all caregivers. Take care of yourself. Some caregivers burn out—it is not easy to watch the process of death. It is not pretty or neat and tidy as it has been depicted in many movies. If you and the patient have decided on home care, plan to take time off and recharge. You should find someone to take your place periodically.

Be realistic about what you and your family can cope with. Take your loved one's needs to heart but factor in your own threshold for stress. And remember, these are stressful times and families tend to bicker when tensions are high, as we said earlier. Having your loved one in an institution can lead to tremendous bouts of guilt and worry as you wonder if he or she is lonely or sad, misses home, is being treated well. Having your loved one at home has its own stresses, and for the person living in the house with the patient, it means never escaping the difficult reality of the situation. Some feel this is a small price to pay for a short time to make a loved one happy in the comfort of their own home, a familiar setting. But for others it is an unbearable burden, and they end up not being able to provide the support they might have been able to if the patient were in a facility. Never be afraid to ask for help.

RESOURCE GUIDE

BOOKS

Family Hospice Care. Harry van Bommel (Scarborough: Resources Supporting Family and Community Legacies Inc., 2002).

This is a must-read for all Canadians, whether they are taking care of a palliative care loved one at this time or not. It will prepare you for the journey ahead, should you confront that situation. (And most of us will.) It provides checklists of the elements you will want to manage if you are helping care for a palliative patient at home. It covers the following topics:

- Hospice care
- Getting organized and making your list
- What to do in an emergency
- What to expect at the end of life
- Managing pain
- Taking care of yourself if you are a caregiver
- Preparing financial and legal affairs
- Preparing funeral arrangements
- Home care tips
- Community resources
- Glossary of terms

Caring for Loved Ones at Home. Harry van Bommel (Scarborough: Resources Supporting Family and Community Legacies Inc., 2002).

This book is not necessarily only about end-of-life care. It is about home care in a more general sense and will help you with topics such as the following:

- Services that can be provided at home
- Adapting your home and getting the right equipment
- Basic care
- How to deal with the care team
- Understanding your condition
- Basic reference guides
- How to find services in your community

Both these books are available for free from the Saint Elizabeth Health Care Foundation website at www.saintelizabeth.com. Saint Elizabeth Health Care has been a sponsor of these publications.

Harry van Bommel has also written other books on care at home, pain, and dying. You can find these by visiting his website at www.legacies.ca.

Let Me Decide: What You Need to Know Now about End-of-Life Care. William Molloy (Toronto: Penguin, 2005).

This short but useful book walks you through the process of filling out your directive. A blank Personal Care Directive is included in the book for the reader to fill in.

ORGANIZATIONS AND ASSOCIATIONS

Canadian Virtual Hospice
www.virtualhospice.ca
This site was created by leading Canadian palliative care experts and will help you access information about end-of-life care and support organizations in Canada related to palliative care. It contains frequently asked questions, offers an opportunity to ask a professional, and provides on-line support. You need to register, but it's easy and the service is free. You can find contact information for hospices and palliative care programs in your area at this site under "Additional Resources."

Dying with Dignity
www.dyingwithdignity.ca
This website will educate patients and caregivers on the rights of individuals as they near the end of life. The organization also provides counselling and information on living wills, advance health care directives, and powers of attorney. It can refer caregivers to a local health care professional with specialized training in end-of-life care.

Canadian Hospice Palliative Care Association
www.chpca.net
This group provides leadership in hospice palliative care, which is aimed at relief of suffering, loneliness, and grief for those who are approaching death.

Living Wills
Joint Centre for Bioethics, University of Toronto
www.jointcentreforbioethics.ca
Blank documents for a living will are available at this website. Click on the Community Tools bar on the lower right and then on "Living Will." This website provides information on how to give legal instructions that allow you to decide which treatment you wish and which you will not permit when you are ill, as well as other instructions for end-of-life care.

CBC News
www.cbc.ca/news/background/wills
CBC News backgrounder: living wills. This site has links to information about living wills and how they are handled in 12 provinces and territories. You will have to complete the disclaimer to have access to this online.

Health Council of Canada
www.healthcouncilcanada.ca
Telephone: (416) 481-7397
This national organization monitors progress that the provinces and territories make in the area of health care reform. It has put together a terrific guide to the Compassionate Care Benefits that can be downloaded from its website. The guide tells you everything you need to know about what the benefit offers and includes a copy of the form you will need to fill out.

Compassionate Care Leave Form
Human Resources and Social Development Canada
Go to the following link and scroll down to the bottom of the page to find the Compassionate Care Benefits Attestation form and information: www.hrsdc.gc.ca/en/ei/types/compassionate_care.shtml.

BOOKSTORES

Many bookstores carry living will kits and forms.

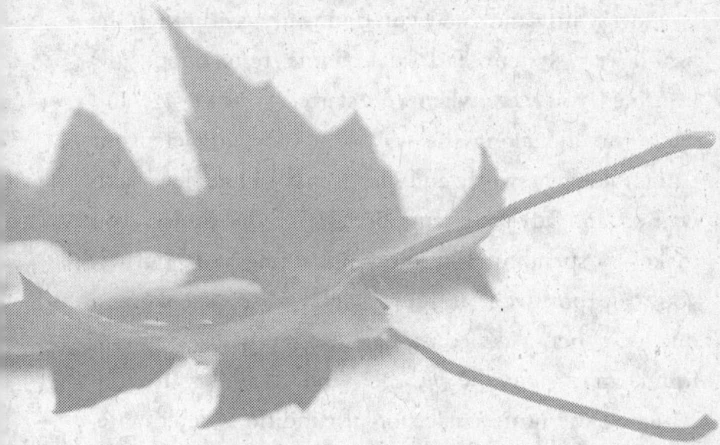

Navigating Care Swiftly and Safely

The success of a patient's voyage can be judged by the swiftness and quality of care obtained. We explore these two dimensions in Chapters 12 and 13. As well, Chapter 14 examines the avenues of complaint open to you and explains how to seek redress if your journey stalls. In sailing, the term "stuck in irons" refers to a sailboat that's stuck facing directly into the wind. Often the boat travels backwards while the skipper struggles to escape. Sometimes a patient care journey gets stuck in irons. Getting moving again is the key to both sailing and patient care. What follows are tips on how to make your journey swifter and safer.

How swiftly and safely you find your way through the health care system and back home rests upon how informed you were when you started your voyage and what you did along the way. You can complete your patient journey swiftly and safely, or have one filled with waiting and adverse events because of the choices you make. By spending a little time planning your journey, you can positively influence its course, speed, and quality. When a skilled captain sets sail with a route in mind, an eye on the weather, and an ability to seek refuge in the nearest safe port if conditions deteriorate, the voyage will be the safest and swiftest. This is also true of your patient journey.

TWELVE

Navigating Canadian Health Care—Swiftly

No single political issue has galvanized Canadian opinion and attention in recent years as much as wait times in the health system. Former Prime Minister Paul Martin made reducing wait times a centrepiece of both his 2004 campaign and his subsequent 10-year plan to fix medicare. Each and every premier and territorial leader signed on to that plan. As part of the plan, $5.5 billion was to be spent over the 10-year period specifically to reduce wait times. This represented some 13 percent of the total increased federal health spending commitment of $41 billion over 10 years. A number of provinces appointed individual leaders to take charge of reducing wait times.

This national policy discussion may seem remote to someone waiting for a new hip or knee or access to an MRI, but it is very relevant to the care you receive and when you receive it. A national mini-industry in analyzing wait times has grown up. There are conferences, special initiatives, advisers, and a frenzy of activity all organized around this topic.

The grand national political debate on health care rivals hockey and the weather as a favourite topic of conversation among Canadians, and it came to a single focus in the early part of the 21st century. Scholars may look back and marvel that in the period from 2000 to 2006, three prime ministers—Jean Chrétien, Paul Martin, and Stephen Harper—grappled with a single issue in health care: how to speed it up. Canadians believed that their health system was not delivering the goods for them. This perception fuelled no fewer than three major federal injections of money into a system that had been cut back in the 1990s. The 10-year plan from 2004 will put $41 billion of new federal spending into provincial coffers.

At the centre of the debate was the frustration of the Canadian public. We have great difficulty judging the exact merits of what we are getting or how long we should be waiting. However, each of us has our own story, about either our own wait in our patient care journey or the wait of a friend or relative. Often these stories take the form of anecdotal evidence about Uncle Fred, who had to go to Buffalo or Minneapolis or Boston to get his MRI because wait times in Canada were too long. These tales, spurred on by a Fraser Institute study that made unflattering comparisons between the number of MRIs in Canada and the number in North Korea, led the federal government in 2000 to invest $1 billion of new money in up-to-the-minute medical technologies. Skilful advocacy from the Canadian Association of Radiologists also played a decisive role. In 2003, another $1.5 billion was committed, all to save Uncle Fred from having to go to Buffalo or Seattle in his quest for an MRI. If you are Uncle Fred, this saga will have more relevance.

In 2004, as noted, $5.5 billion was allocated over a number of years to reduce wait times for the "Big Five" tests or surgeries: cancer surgery, heart surgery, diagnostic imaging, joint replacement, and vision restoration. These areas are of most concern to aging boomers as well as the elderly. The provinces and the Government of Canada agreed to measure wait times in each of these areas so they could see where—and how much—improvement was needed. Statistics Canada surveyed Canadians about their access. Each and every government in Canada undertook work; the Canadian Medical Association organized a Wait Times Coalition, which produced its own detailed plan to reduce wait times.

Even the Supreme Court of Canada weighed in on this issue in 2005 in the case of a patient, George Zeliotis, and his physician, Dr. Jacques Chaoulli. The court ruling signalled to all governments that the public health system must deliver timely care or the courts will open the door to a private system. The Supreme Court judgment means that governments have to do more to reduce wait times. They have to make measurable progress. This decision proved to be a profound wake-up call for the provinces and the health delivery system.

In the wake of the Supreme Court decision, Paul Martin appointed Dr. Brian Postl, CEO of the Winnipeg Regional Health Authority, as the federal adviser on wait times. During the election campaign of 2006, both Paul Martin and Stephen Harper endorsed "care guarantees" as a means to ensure that those waiting too long could get access to speedier care. Timely access to care—navigating the health care system swiftly—has clearly become the issue of the day. Concrete action and investments in the care system are speeding up access.

What does all this mean for you? First, it likely means that wait times will be reduced over the coming years. Second, it means that for particular procedures, you will be able to get information about wait times at various hospitals more easily and therefore seek treatment in a location with the shortest waiting list. Third, in an extreme case, there may be more responsiveness from the health system, from governments, and from various appeal panels to a complaint based on the length of time you're waiting. This issue is covered in depth in Chapter 14.

Some things don't change, though. With health care, as with many other facets of human life—whether it's getting a ticket to a sporting event, a good table at the right restaurant, or a flight using your Aeroplan miles—the more knowledgeable you are about how the system works and how the game is played, the better you can do.

Five Tools for Timely Care

What can you do as an individual citizen to ensure that your patient care journey is carried out as swiftly as possible? We have suggestions that will help you get faster care—you will recognize some of the themes from earlier chapters. We've organized them under five broad headings: information, advocacy, self-management, networking, and appropriateness.

1. Information

Information is power. You need to become as informed as possible about where to go for care.

Plenty of information is now being released by health care organizations and governments so you will know where care is slow and where care is fast. This information is often available on websites that can help guide you to a swifter health care journey. You need to find it and then use it to improve your own access. You should also look for information from news stories or from your doctor about hospitals or clinics with fast service. Learn how to find the speedy places for care and gain access to them. Learn how to ask those questions or position yourself in ways that can speed your journey along more quickly. A simple question should be posed to your physician or surgeon at the time your treatment or diagnosis is first discussed: "Is there a faster way?"

Here's an example from Michael's experience again. A colonoscopy done on a very close friend revealed something that looked like colon cancer. The necessary confirming test was an ultrasound, and because colon cancer is generally slow growing, the specialist proposed an ultrasound a week or 10 days later. Michael asked the specialist whether it was possible to get an ultrasound the same day and was told that if Michael and his friend went quickly across the city, to a particular clinic, they would be the first there when it opened. The specialist's office called at 8 A.M. to let the doctor in charge of the ultrasound clinic know they would be coming. This simple question netted an ultrasound and a diagnosis within hours of the original colonoscopy, rather than days, weeks, or months later.

These are the essential tactics to get you started on a faster journey and below are some tips to help you further.

The Canadian Institute for Health Information (www.cihi.ca) recently published a report entitled *Waiting for Health Care in Canada—What We Know and What We Don't Know*, which has a wealth of information. It's a big-picture report, but most Canadians aren't interested in the big picture, particularly when they or someone they care about is ill. They're interested in a very small picture—the small picture of how they are going to get care and get it quickly.

You can make use of studies like this, though. For example, this report noted that for hip and knee replacements, nearly one-third of the time that elapses between the referral to a specialist and getting the surgery is spent waiting for the initial visit to the orthopedic surgeon. Anything you can do to speed up your visit to the orthopedic surgeon could shave as much as a third off the total wait time. How do you go about trying to shave some time off that long wait? You can take a number of concrete steps to shorten your wait time. First, because referral letters are sometimes lost, ask for a copy and convey it yourself to the specialist's office. While you are delivering the letter, chat with the nurse or receptionist and seek an early appointment. Often if you are willing to come in early or late or be available if someone cancels, you can get seen faster. Let's look at the data from CIHI on hip fractures and see what we can learn from it. In the year 2003–2004, 24,000 Canadians were admitted for surgery following a broken hip. Thirty-one percent had their surgery the same day they were admitted and 41 percent had it the next day, and yet 16 percent waited two days, 6 percent three days, and 6 percent four or more days. The CIHI data established that the size of the hospital mattered. The larger the hospital, the less likely it was that the patient had his or her hip repaired the same day. One point to be gleaned from the data is that you may get faster service by going to a smaller hospital. But there is a tradeoff between speed and quality. The best advice is to go to the smaller local hospital for smaller operations or more routine matters. If you are facing complex surgery, as Chapter 13 makes clear, you want a bigger place that does lots of volume of that particular procedure. Ask your doctor for advice on this question.

In December 2005, provincial health ministers set a goal that hip fracture operations should take place within 48 hours of admittance. One in four Canadians waits longer for this surgery. Knowing that health ministers have set this standard is valuable information. It allows you to ask at the time of admission whether the hospital is meeting this standard. This alone may be an important point of leverage to accelerate care. And it's clear that there are better ways of doing things. For example, the Alberta Bone and Joint Institute in Calgary has reduced its wait time for joint replacement from 47 weeks to 4.7 weeks—you might want to be referred there rather than to the congested and less organized part of the system. This time saving came about because improvements were made to how the process was organized—the patient is better informed, the nurses can spend more time assisting the patient, and the surgeon concentrates on doing what he or she does best: the surgery.

At the micro-level, each patient's journey is unique. It's that uniqueness that offers the possibility of quicker service. Getting care swiftly is a matter of doing some homework to determine where care will be delivered more rapidly. As we said earlier, many hospitals and health regions within Canada post wait times for particular procedures on the Internet. The day we searched the wait times site established by Ontario's ministry of health, we found that the median wait time for cataract surgery in Toronto was 69 days at St. Michael's Hospital and 169 days at Sunnybrook Health Sciences Centre.

In some cases, wait times are consolidated so you get the first available specialist. But often this is not the case. You may need to intervene and point out to your family doctor that from material gleaned on the Internet you know that a referral to hospital A might produce a much shorter wait than a referral to hospital B. Your physician may well push back and explain that his or her reason for preferring hospital B is that the hospital has greater expertise in the area in which you need care. Better quality is certainly a valid reason to wait longer. But in many cases, your doctor may just be uninformed about wait times. Do some more research to see if the standard is higher in hospital B. Some hospitals publish outcome data, but the major source is the Canadian Institute for Health Information (www.cihi.ca). By taking responsibility for your patient care journey, you can accelerate that journey.

Tips

Look for stories about faster care. Innovators in faster care tend to attract news coverage.

Consult the wait time websites listed in the Resource Guide at the end of this chapter.

Ask about standard wait time targets at your hospital. All this information can help you as you complete your journey.

2. Advocacy

The second tool is advocacy. Advocacy gets faster care. Become an advocate for yourself, and then identify allies who will be your advocates and tap into their clout. If you want timely care for yourself or a loved one, it is a good idea to make plain why you want it and what the beneficial consequences would be both for the person getting the care and for society. Most frequently advocates are friends or relatives who can speak up on your behalf if you're too tired or weak or temporarily confused—or just plain scared!

Tip

Find a forceful person among your family or friends and ask him or her to serve as your advocate.

One type of advocacy can be seen in the fact that the Canada Health Act specifically excludes Workers' Compensation Boards from its rules. There was a simple reason for this: The founders of the Canada Health Act and medicare wanted Workers' Compensation Boards to be able to get faster care for injured workers. Getting injured workers back to work rapidly helps the solvency of the Workers' Compensation Boards, the performance of the Canadian workforce, and most important, the long-term health of the injured workers. There is plenty of evidence that injured workers, particularly those with soft tissue injuries, do much better if they get rapid rehabilitation. If rehabilitation is delayed, a back or knee or other part of the human body can stiffen, and an injured worker can become a permanently disabled worker. This result has enormous consequences for you and an enormous cost to the Workers' Compensation Board.

Here's another example of advocacy: Mats Sundin, the captain of the Toronto Maple Leafs, was carted off the ice not long ago for an almost instantaneous MRI and was back, pronounced fit to play, by the third period. Michael was asked, "How does he get a fast MRI when my cousin Joe can't?" Our only reply is that it may not be fair, but 20,000 Leafs fans roared their approval at Sundin's return. There are only so many hockey games in a season and so many seasons in a hockey player's career. These players get rapid access because they are important assets to their team. The team owners and managers are, in effect, the advocates for each player. Many employers have entered into arrangements of various sorts with local hospitals or physicians to try to get faster care for their employees. Although Canadian workers are not facing an arena filled with cheering fans, they are important to their employers when they are able to do a full and top-quality day's work. Their return to health is also important to their families, who depend upon them.

Both your employer and the Workers' Compensation Board can be important advocates for you depending on your circumstances. If you have been injured in an automobile accident, the insurer may be an advocate for access to rehabilitative care. Some major corporations have their own health professionals, such as company doctors and nurses. They may be a good first stop if you are not getting rapid access to care.

Tip

Advocate for yourself with people and organizations that can help. You have allies in your employer and your insurers; both want to get you quick access and a return to work and health—use them to help.

Michael's father was a busy orthopedic surgeon at the Manitoba Clinic in Winnipeg. As a child, Michael would watch and learn how his father's office operated. It was always busy and yet there was always an opportunity to slide in an extra-urgent patient or someone who just needed to get the attention of the surgeon. How was this done? Well, in that office control rested with the nurse. She managed the patient flow in the office and the booking and rebooking of appointments and tests. In particular, she could slide someone in either at the beginning of the afternoon of appointments or at the end. That nurse was the person you needed to be on the best terms with. She had the power to grant access.

Tip

Whether it's a nurse, a secretary, or an administrative assistant, find the person who does the booking. These people can be great allies if you get to know them.

It's not always easy to be cheerful and friendly when you're not feeling well or you're worried about the health of someone close to you. But if you are an angry, demanding, rude patient, it is not likely you'll impress the nurse or office manager, and that in turn may make her reluctant to go to extra trouble to get you in early. On the other hand, if you show some thoughtfulness and indicate clearly the reasons why an earlier visit would be advantageous, you have a much greater chance of getting seen. In every busy physician's office, there are cancellations. One tactic Michael has employed on more than one occasion is simply to offer to make himself immediately available should a cancellation arise. The combination of being on good terms with the surgeon or physician's nurse or assistant and being willing to turn up on very short notice can often accelerate entry. Your family doctor can be a powerful advocate for earlier care as well.

Tip

Advocate with your doctors. Enlist their support. They can sometimes get you in faster if you show how important it is to you.

3. Self-Management

The third tool is the control and management of your own patient care journey. Only you can really determine the tactics and strategies you are willing to engage to improve the speed of your care.

Perhaps the most telling example of the dual realities that can often exist in health care came one day in 1999 for Michael, who was spending the day chairing a conference on health care. The focus of the conference was largely on the wait times issue. Key topics included the lack of physicians, particularly specialists, as well as the nursing shortage. Several speakers made rather broad and sweeping comments about the impossibility of accessing a specialist on a timely basis.

At various breaks for coffee and lunch, Michael was engaged in an ongoing and urgent cellphone conversation with his teenage daughter, Geneviève. Michael recounts the story:

> Geneviève had refused to attend school that morning, a situation I was alerted to by her high school. When I reached Geneviève at home, she was in tears. After consoling her, I learned that her reason for not going to school was that her chin had turned bright red. She was determined not to face the embarrassment her bright red chin would cause for her in a school setting. When her tears subsided, Geneviève let me know that her condition had likely been caused by one of five medications her dermatologist had prescribed for her acne. She had already been busy on the Internet tracking down information on each of the drugs. She had narrowed the field to two suspects that could possibly cause that side effect.
>
> Her story unfolded throughout the day as I called her on breaks from the doom and gloom of the

> conference with its repeated statements that "nobody could get timely access to a specialist." By noon she had been in touch with her dermatologist's office, and had learned that he was en route to a conference in California and was changing planes in Chicago. She convinced his office to give her his cellphone number, and she contacted him in Chicago. After a brief discussion, they agreed which of the acne drugs she should suspend. Their joint work caused her chin to go back to its normal colour. The next day she was willing and able to go back to school.

To Michael, there was a stark contrast between one view of the health care system, the old historic view that access meant visits by a patient to a doctor or hospital, and a more modern definition of access that unbundled the information from the visit. In the old world of health care, all information was held by the physician and obtaining information always involved a visit. In the modern digital world of health care, this information monopoly is gone. As a consequence, health information and care decisions have detached themselves from the office visit. They have been "unbundled." Michael's daughter had been able to find important information on the Internet and then, taking charge of her situation, had advocated on her own behalf, which resulted in a telephone conversation with her dermatologist, who agreed on a course of action. She had the access she needed virtually in real time, on the same day, to get done what she needed to get done. If her request to the dermatologist's office had been for an appointment, she likely would have waited several weeks, particularly since the condition she described, a bright red chin, would not have been seen as one causing any threat to her continuing health or life. It's possible that she could have waited one or several weeks if she had chosen the more passive role; instead, she got same-day service.

There are obvious limitations to the unbundling of care from the visit, but in a surprising number of cases at least some part of the patient care journey can be managed without a visit to the doctor. Rather, the visit could be to a particular part of the health care system such as a pharmacy. (In many larger centres some pharmacies are open 24 hours a day). In addition, a

Tip

Not all health advice and assistance requires a visit to the doctor. Hospitals and governments are hard at work creating settings for less urgent patients. Even where these have been created, Canadians are still drawn to the large white H of the hospital. It remains a beacon of hope. But what are some of the available alternatives? Family health teams, community health centres, and urgent care clinics that offer 24-hour, seven-day-a-week care are not yet the standard across Canada, but they are expanding steadily. If you join one of these reformed primary care groups as a patient, you will gain access to care at off hours. In addition to primary care groups, there are urgent care clinics at some hospitals. Or try a call to the 1-800 nurse call line in your province before a visit to the emergency department. You may find that the information you need is accessible by telephone without a visit.

number of hospitals have created urgent care clinics to take the pressure off their emergency rooms. You may need to consult a nurse call line to decide the appropriate place to go. If you have severe chest pain or other major symptoms, go to the emergency department. If you have a bad cold or flu, then the urgent care clinic is a better option. Err on the side of caution, but don't go to the emergency department just out of habit.

Many wait lists are badly kept or not kept at all. Often, those who are patient and responsible suffer, because the ball is dropped between their referring physician's office and the specialist's office. The patient is at home waiting for a call from the specialist. But the specialist's office is never going to make that call because they've lost the letter from the referring physician, or the staff has changed, or any one of a hundred other things have happened. It is vitally important that you *manage every step*. If your doctor is referring you to a specialist, ask your doctor's office when the referral letter went and, even better, if it is possible to obtain a copy of that letter. You then need to follow up with the specialist and make sure your appointment is being scheduled on a timely basis. You are dealing with a big system, a paper-based system, and frankly things get lost. Patient records, diagnostic tests, and referral letters go missing.

Another aspect of this paper-based system is that when you show up at a specialist's office, they more often than not have no information about you, other than your physical presence. This oversight results in a lot of duplicate testing. It can also delay your treatment. It is important—if you can possibly make it happen—that your test results go along with you to the receiving doctor. It is even better if those results have been sent on ahead. With electronic patient records, this will become an easier process. But at the moment, you can play a role by getting a copy of everything.

Tip

Pay attention to the details of your journey, particularly the referrals. Organize to ensure each step proceeds as swiftly as possible.

Michael has another story about his daughter, Geneviève, that illustrates how you can take self-management a step farther or approach it from a slightly different angle.

> A number of years ago, when she was young, my daughter, Geneviève, fell on a family snowboarding vacation near Vernon, British Columbia. I took her into the Vernon hospital, suspecting from the degree of pain she was exhibiting that she had probably broken her wrist. I went with Geneviève and the X-ray technician as he X-rayed her wrist. We then sat in the emergency department waiting room hoping for the result. After a while, I realized how short-staffed the hospital emergency department was. After a pleasant conversation with the nurse, I learned that the X-ray had been developed but was at the far end of the hospital. No porter or staff

member had the time to go down to get it. I volunteered to make the trip myself in this small hospital. I believe that largely because they were understaffed and I was friendly and came across as a concerned father, not as an impatient or angry father, they were pleased to accept my offer of assistance. I walked the length of the hospital, found the X-ray department, spoke with the technician, and returned to the emergency room with the X-ray. I don't know if I violated any rules of the hospital in this, but I was concerned with getting my daughter's treatment underway without further waiting. The X-ray was examined by the busy emergency department doctor. He pronounced that she did in fact have a break of her wrist but it was undisplaced—that is, the bone hadn't moved. Therefore the damage could be treated with a simple cast. The cast was put on and we were back to the ski resort in time to join the others for dinner.

When we were leaving the Vernon hospital, it occurred to me to ask the X-ray technician if we could get a copy of her X-ray and he agreed. Back in Toronto, Geneviève and I went to see an orthopedic surgeon at the Toronto Western Hospital to find out when the cast should be removed. I brought along the X-ray. He told her to come back in three weeks and he would take the cast off. As we were leaving, he handed me back the X-ray. I said, "Shouldn't you keep that X-ray for her file?" He said, "You care more about it. We'll probably lose it. You keep it." He communicated to me a true but often overlooked reality: As a patient or a family member of a patient, you care a great deal about that information.

Tip

Volunteer to help. Don't just sit there waiting.

It's not that your hospital doesn't care; it's just that it's a large system. This orthopedist was probably just signalling his own frustration that records went missing. If at all possible, you should obtain duplicates of important test results and keep them, as previously noted in this book, in a personal health record file.

Another less happy tale occurred the day that Michael accompanied his brother-in-law through a whole battery of ultrasounds, blood tests, and so on for a very serious cancer he was battling. Hospitals are remarkably complex organizations. Even though both men were extremely knowledgeable about the health system, they waited for a considerable period of time for the ultrasound. The delay meant a return trip the next day for the blood tests. Later a doctor Michael knows in the hospital asked, "Why didn't you go and get the blood tests done while you were waiting for the ultrasound?"

This was a very good question that they hadn't thought to ask. A complex system like a hospital can often generate waiting not out of design but simply out of the normal complexities. A few well-asked questions—"Can I fetch the X-ray? Could we get the blood test done while we're waiting for the ultrasound?"—can often speed a patient's journey.

4. Networking

The fourth tool is your network. Personal connection goes a long way. The difference between networking and advocacy is what you are seeking. With an advocate you are seeking a voice and support. With networking you are seeking information and access. It is not impossible that someone in your network might become your advocate, but it is not essential. Today and every day in Canada over 1 million people get out of their beds and go to work in the health care system. It is unlikely that you are very far removed from someone who is part of that enormous workforce. Your aunt may be a nurse, your cousin may be a doctor, or your sister may be a lab technician—each of them has connections to the health system and may have some ability to help you attain swifter care.

When it comes to health care for most Canadians, we are talking not of six degrees of separation, but of one or two. In nearly every family there is someone with some connection to the health system. All of those people can be allies in your quest for quicker care. Any one of them may have a relationship with someone who could give them advice about how you might get faster access to care. Often people in the health care system are only too eager to help out. After all, the vast majority of them work in the health system because it is a calling and offers an opportunity to do some good in the world. Just as having a brother-in-law who's an auto mechanic can be helpful to the health of your automobile, having a relative who is inside the health system may be very useful to you in ensuring your own care or the care of a loved one.

Another avenue is to follow the patient journey of a friend. If your friend has been through surgery of one sort or another and found the surgeon thoughtful as well as competent, he or she may be willing to make an introduction. Physicians, like others, are subject to the human desire to be appreciated. An appreciative former patient calling a doctor to ask if he or she would be willing to see a friend or loved one with the same condition will usually be met with a positive response. You may recognize some similarities in our suggestions about how to treat the large health care system and the way you would go shopping. The shopping analogy generally offends people in health care, but there are aspects of it that are applicable. If you got terrific service at a store, you are inclined to recommend it to your friends. If you got terrific service at a hospital, it is equally reasonable to assume that you might recommend it.

Tip

Make a list of friends and family who work in the health system for that day in the future when you might need to ask for help.

5. Appropriateness

The fifth tool is to ask yourself whether you really need care at all. Appropriateness is a critical consideration. Can you really get the right outcome if you speed up access to the wrong care? Do you have alternatives to the care you think you need?

Keep in mind that sometimes the care you seek is not the care you need. Let me give a couple of illustrations of this. A cousin of mine, a young law student faced with back surgery to deal with incredible and debilitating lower back pain, phoned my father to get a second opinion. My surgeon father, while willing to see him, asked him several questions before subjecting my cousin to plane travel from Vancouver to Winnipeg. He asked about his daily routine. My cousin replied that he lived on the ocean and ran five miles on the hard-packed sand of the beach every morning.

My father's advice was, "Stop running on the beach."

The pain subsided and my cousin never required the surgery that would have left him with a permanent stiffness in his lower back.

Here's another simple illustration. An overweight woman had had both hips replaced. While she was waiting for knee-replacement surgery, she experienced a dramatic loss of weight, probably 100 or more pounds. The result was that the knee surgery was no longer necessary. There are alternatives to surgery that may get you the result without the waiting or the risks of the surgery itself.

Tip

Even after you are scheduled for surgery, there are steps you can take to reduce risk and improve outcome. The world-famous Shouldice Clinic weighs patients seeking hernia repair (its specialty). It sets a date and a target weight. If you do not reach the target weight, you do not get the surgery. Why? Risk! By reaching the target weight, you reduce your risk of a bad outcome.

What Governments Are Doing to Improve Wait Times

As noted, in an effort to respond to the demands of the public, governments across the country are cajoling, bribing, and reorganizing physicians and other health care providers into teams and networks. Most provinces have a service that gives you phone access to a highly qualified nurse with 10 years or more of experience. (The numbers for the various jurisdictions are listed in the Resource Guide at the end of this chapter.) These nurses can work with you to sort out the condition you're faced with, advising you on whether you should be going to the emergency department of your hospital or waiting to be treated the next day in a physician's office. Nurses on call lines can also make very helpful suggestions about what you can do to manage the symptoms of the condition you're dealing with.

In western Canada many of the health regions have introduced methods to better coordinate care. Not only have they posted wait times on their websites, but they are endeavouring to create organized wait lists. Saskatchewan is using an overall surgical wait list for all patients in that province. All patients are assessed by their doctor for the urgency of their case, and a score is assigned. The process is transparent to patients. Their own description of their circumstances, such as pain or difficulty in moving, determines that score. The province has been able to chop the tail end of the wait times from several years to at maximum 18 months. Eighteen months is still a long time for some types of surgery, particularly joint replacement, but it is a vast improvement for those patients who have been waiting in excess of two years. More detail of this program can be found at www.sasksurgery.ca.

Wait times are measured in two ways—one is the average wait time; the other is the time for those waiting the longest, the so-called tail. Getting 80 percent of all cases done in two weeks may be terrific, but not if the remaining 20 percent of patients are left to wait months or years.

Innovative efforts are being made to improve overall wait times in various parts of Canada. Just as clinical trials for new drugs are worth considering as treatment, so are pilot programs that may speed up your access to care.

How to Locate Information on Wait Times

A starting point on tracking down faster care is to get on the Internet. The chart on the next page shows how to get information from each of the 10 provinces on wait times for particular services.

SURFING FOR WAIT TIMES

All provinces provide some wait-time data on websites or in reports, but the scope and depth of reporting varies considerably. The level of detail also differs and is changing rapidly. The following table shows which jurisdictions reported some wait-time information as of December 2005 and lists the websites where this information can be accessed.

Posting wait times is an evolving field. You will note that some provinces provide information on only one or

	Websites with Wait-Time Information Go the Health Canada homepage: www.hc-sc.gc.ca, English. Select Index A–Z, then select: Wait Times in Canada. Scroll down to Provincial and Territorial Province Initiatives, or go to these individual sites:
NS	www.gov.ns.ca/health/waittimes/wt_treatment_service/default.htm
NB	www1.gnb.ca/0217/surgicalwaittimes/Reports/index-e.aspx
QC	wpp01.msss.gouv.qc.ca/appl/g74web/
ON	www.health.gov.on.ca/transformation/wait_times/public/wt_public_mn.html
MB	www.gov.mb.ca/health/waittime/index.html?/index.html
SK	www.sasksurgery.ca/wait-list-info.htm
AB	www.ahw.gov.ab.ca/waitlist/WaitListPublicHome.jsp
BC	www.healthservices.gov.bc.ca/waitlist/index.html

two of the priority areas, while others are more comprehensive. It's worth noting that this information was current as of December 2005, and these websites are under continual evaluation or in some cases expansion. Individual health regions and individual hospitals also provide detailed reporting on wait times. Just as you can determine whether your Air Canada flight is on time or delayed without making a phone call, you can now determine whether hip replacement is faster in Calgary or Edmonton or Saskatoon.

Organized Care Networks

A new type of network, called an organized care network, is emerging in parts of the country and parts of health care service, particularly complex surgeries. The leading program in Canada is the Cardiac Care Network (CCN) of Ontario (www.ccn.on.ca). The CCN is a fully organized system of care for the thousands of heart surgery patients passing through the system each year. Here's how it works: Patients are assessed on an urgency score, and then based on the scores, regional coordinators help plan and organize the care journey. A computerized registry prevents patients from falling between the cracks. Patients can choose to go on a waiting list for a particular surgeon or accept the next available surgeon. Research and monitoring has allowed for a high standard of care across all cardiac surgeons in Ontario. This solves the problem of one surgeon having a very small waiting list while others have very long lists. The pooling of the waiting lists significantly reduces wait times for everyone. If you live in Ontario and require cardiac surgery, you should automatically be informed of this practice.

Variations of this network method are emerging in other parts of the country. The Ontario Cardiac Care Network is seen by many experts as a model for what will develop for many types of complex surgery to shorten wait times and simultaneously improve quality. As a patient, you should find out whether your province or health region has an organized system for managing wait lists.

Throughout the health care system, goverments are making massive investments to speed care. To benefit, though, you need to be the master and the manager of your patient care journey. Asking the right questions during your journey is essential. The timely question mid-journey can mean an invisible roadblock to quick care is circumvented.

RESOURCE GUIDE

PATIENT ADVOCACY AND NAVIGATION

NavaHealth Inc.
http://navahealth.ca
info@navahealth.ca
Telephone: (604) 269-2426 or 1-866-591-6282

Qualicare Inc.
www.qualicare.ca
info@qualicare.ca
Telephone: (416) 630-0202

ORGANIZATIONS AND ASSOCIATIONS

Canadian Institute for Health Information
www.cihi.ca
This site can give you access to the report entitled *Waiting for Health Care in Canada—What We Know and What We Don't Know*, which has a wealth of information. This is a good report for those interested in the big picture.

PROVINCIAL WAIT-TIMES WEBSITES

As well as consulting the provincial websites, check the health authorities and hospitals in your area to see if they post wait-time data to their own websites. The list below is not comprehensive. If your province is not covered below, start with your local hospital or provincial department of health website.

Ontario
www.health.gov.on.ca
This website has a search function for wait times. You can compare wait times for cataract surgery, diagnostics, cancer, joint replacement, and heart surgery at all the hospitals in your city.

Manitoba
www.gov.mb.ca
Manitoba Health provides wait-time data by hospital for the five key areas. It also provides data on volumes of surgery.

Saskatchewan
www.sasksurgery.ca
This site is mostly geared to surgery wait times. It has a very thoughtful section entitled "Moving through the System." Even if you are not a resident of Saskatchewan, the step-by-step description of the surgical process is an informative read.

Nova Scotia
www.gov.ns.ca
This site links to a wait-times site. There is good information on cancer and other specialist services.

The Western Canada Wait List Project
www.wcwl.org/
This project undertook a great deal of work on wait times and standards in western Canada. Its website is a good source of information on this subject.

Telephone Services for Health Information and Advice
Nurse call lines have been established in many parts of Canada. They are free; open 24 hours a day, seven days a week; confidential; and staffed by experienced registered nurses. The following listing will help you access this valuable service.

Ontario Telehealth
Telephone: 1-866-797-0000

B.C. Nurseline
Telephone: 1-866-215-4700
The B.C. service also has a pharmacist on call from 5 P.M. each day to 9 A.M. the next day.

Health Link Alberta
Telephone: (403) 943-5465 (Calgary)
Telephone: (780) 408-5465 (Edmonton)
Toll-free 1-866-408-5465 (elsewhere)

Info-Santé (Quebec)
Telephone: (514) 934-0354

Saskatchewan HealthLine
Telephone: 1-877-800-0002

New Brunswick TeleCare
Telephone: 1-800-244-8353

Manitoba HealthLinks
Telephone: 1-888-315-9257 (limited service)

Newfoundland and Labrador has announced a telenurse service, but it is not yet available. Nova Scotia and Prince Edward Island do not offer this service.

THIRTEEN

Navigating Canadian Health Care—Safely

It is difficult to navigate the Canadian health care system successfully. It is also difficult to get access to the health care services you need. Even when you navigate skilfully and gain access, your challenges are not over. You also need to navigate the health care system safely!

You may ask, "How dangerous can health care be? Surely it is the absence of health care that threatens our health. Surely it is disease and injuries that threaten our well-being." This is true. It is also true that overwhelmingly the health care system does more good than harm. However, recent studies conclude that the health care system is far from a safe place. When you step into a Canadian hospital as a patient, you have a 1 in 13 chance of experiencing an adverse event!

The Institute of Medicine in the United States found in 2000 that nearly 100,000 deaths per year in that country were the result of avoidable errors. This ranked adverse events as the eighth-highest cause of death in the United States, ahead of AIDS, breast cancer, and motor vehicle accidents.

The most thorough study of patient safety in hospitals across Canada was led by Professor Ross Baker at the University of Toronto and Dr. Peter Norton. The Baker-Norton study, published in May 2004, showed that the Canadian health care system is like health care systems in other nations: error prone. Baker and Norton found that each year the Canadian hospital system, in dealing with 2.5 million admissions, produces 185,000 adverse events, of which 75,000 are preventable. These adverse events lead to between 9250 and 23,750 preventable patient deaths. This is the equivalent of a fully loaded commercial airliner crashing with 200 passengers on board every week. Fortunately, air travel has become so safe that in some years in Canada there are no fatalities, even though millions of Canadians fly every year. Millions of Canadians also use the health care system every year, and sadly it is not nearly as safe as flying. Perhaps it never can be fully as safe as flying, but it can be much safer than it is now.

A lot of careful work is beginning to improve the safety of the health care system. The Canadian Patient Safety Institute, which was founded in Edmonton a few years ago, is undertaking a number of projects to make the health care system safer in Canada.

Tip

The Canadian Patient Safety Institute has a website you can visit for tips on patient safety: www.patientsafetyinstitute.ca.

But despite the best efforts of this institute and others like it, there is no guarantee that your patient care journey will be as safe as you'd like it to be. Only you, armed with knowledge and information, can take steps to at least minimize some of the most serious threats to your safety.

Much research has focused on the sources of adverse events in recent years. A decade ago this whole field was called "medical error," a term that implied that these errors were all the result of mistakes made by doctors. A sponge left inside the wound after closure in surgery or a wrong drug prescribed were classic examples. A more thoughtful look at the situation convinced researchers that for catastrophic outcomes to occur, a series of mistakes need to be made. A single error is usually corrected. A catastrophic result is certainly not the sole fault of bad doctors or of good doctors making a mistake on a particular day. This insight has shaped efforts to change the health culture so that errors are acknowledged and corrected. It has also led to work on processes to reduce the potential for errors.

One remarkable success story is worth commenting upon because it demonstrates how much improvement can be achieved with a determined effort. Thirty years ago the anaesthetics given to most patients facing major surgery resulted in 1 death for every 3500 anaesthetics administered. A determined effort by organized anaesthesiology has resulted in a dramatic improvement. Not only do anaesthesiologists now pay much lower malpractice premiums, but the fatality rate has dropped to 1 in 350,000. That's right—anaesthesiology is 100 times safer than it was 30 years ago! This is not true of the health care system as a whole, but it is the example that demonstrates the potential for improvement.

Why was anaesthesiology able to achieve this triumph of quality improvement? The determined effort included not only better training but redesigning the process of anaesthesia itself so that it was much more difficult for an error to be made. For example, fittings in operating rooms were changed so that the wrong gas could not be hooked up, a common source of earlier errors and fatalities. Most important, anaesthesia has created a culture of safety and quality improvement.

Safer Health Care Now

In 2005, the "Safer Healthcare Now" campaign was launched, backed by the Canadian Patient Safety Institute and over 80 health care organizations. At the heart of the campaign are six strategies targeted at the leading sources of adverse outcomes and avoidable deaths for patients. These are the areas where the evidence shows potential to reduce deaths.

Six Areas to Target to Reduce Adverse Effects

This list is useful to you as a patient or an advocate for a patient because it provides a roadmap of some of the danger zones. Most of these are items requiring action by your care team and are directed to the medical community. However, patients will benefit from knowing about these goals as it will make them aware of where problems are most often encountered in the patient care journey. We have added some translation of the health care vocabulary.

1. Organizing rapid response teams to deal with early signs of patient decline in hospital settings outside intensive care. In other words, when a patient's condition worsens, rapid action is essential and there should be a team ready to deal with it immediately.
2. Preventing avoidable deaths from heart attacks through more consistent evidenced-based care. Many heart disease patients do not get the medication they require. Make certain that the necessary medications are prescribed and taken. An Ontario study by the Institute for Clinical Evaluative Sciences (ICES) reports that a single Aspirin taken each day after a heart attack could save hundreds of lives in Ontario alone. You should ask your family doctor, your cardiologist (heart specialist), and your pharmacist for their advice on the best

drugs to manage your heart condition.

3. Preventing adverse drug events by better reconciliation of medications. You can help in this area by keeping your own list of your medications. It also helps if you go to the same pharmacy to fill prescriptions so the pharmacist can monitor for interaction among your medications. Ensure that your family doctor is updated on all medications, particularly those prescribed by others.
4. Preventing central line infections. Here you are relying on the hospital staff to do a conscientious job in cleaning medical equipment used to give intravenous treatments. You should be alert for any signs of infection, such as a fever.
5. Preventing surgical site infections by reliably delivering antibiotics before, during, and after surgery and other evidenced-based care at the proper time. Hospitals are dangerous places. A significant number of patients develop infections while in hospital. As a patient, you should watch carefully for signs such as a fever that could indicate an infection. Ask to be informed of any antibiotics needed to combat potential infections. In a hospital these antibiotics are often administered through the intravenous line into your arm.
6. Preventing ventilator-associated pneumonia through organized ventilator protocols. In other words, pneumonia can be avoided by following the rules for treatment when using a ventilator. When

a patient is on a ventilator—a machine that breathes for the patient—pneumonia can be a complication because the patient is not able to be upright or move around, and thus cannot clear his or her lungs. To prevent pneumonia from developing, the nursing and medical staff should follow the steps recommended for using the equipment.

These six goals are important to improving safety in the hospital system, as well as in the home and community. Most of the steps to achieve these goals can be put into action only by medical caregivers. However, there are other strategies you need to pursue.

Five Key Steps You Can Take to Ensure a Safer Journey

Here are things that you can do to improve the safety of your own patient care journey or the journey of your friends and family.

1. Get to the right place—where you receive care is important.
2. Know your drugs—avoid medication errors.
3. Have the right care team—know exactly who is caring for you.
4. Know your chronic disease—manage it.
5. Do not go alone—bring an advocate.

Let's consider each of these ideas in more detail.

1. Get to the Right Place

Where you get care is important. Much research has focused on the connections between volumes of surgeries and outcomes from surgery. An old cliché sums up the results: Practice makes perfect. In complex health care, practice certainly makes for better care. For complex procedures, such as heart surgery, complex cancer surgery, and other highly involved procedures, the evidence is overwhelming: Having your procedure done somewhere where they do a lot of the same procedure will get you a better result. This does not mean that for every medical procedure, you should rush off to a centre with high volumes. Many simple procedures can be done routinely and safely close to your home, in your local doctor's office or your local hospital. Most ordinary procedures can be done with a reasonable degree of safety and no significant difference in outcome. But this is not the case for more complex surgeries.

Residents of Winnipeg learned this truth in a tragic fashion. The Health Science Centre in Winnipeg began a pediatric cardiovascular surgery program in 1994—heart surgeries for babies and infants. The results were disastrous. Twelve babies died following surgery. The program was finally halted in 1995, when nurses refused to attend in the operating room.

A judicial inquiry was called. Judge Murray Sinclair investigated the sources of the high fatality rates among those babies operated on. The inquiry heard from 86 witnesses over a 31-month period and produced 48,000 pages of transcripts. Judge Sinclair concluded that the deaths were primarily the result of a mismatch between the cases selected and the skills of the single surgeon hired for the program. In many respects, it was the low volume of procedures that didn't allow for a fully skilled team of surgeons qualified to do the full range of heart surgery procedures. As a consequence of the recommendations of the Sinclair Inquiry, the Government of Manitoba agreed to shift all Manitoba heart surgery on infants to the Children's Hospital in Edmonton, Alberta, where sufficient volumes would support good outcomes. Other western provinces have joined in this high-quality

Tip

If you are facing a major surgery, particularly a complex surgery, find out whether the hospital you are being referred to does a sufficient volume of these procedures to get you a good outcome. For complex procedures, you don't want to be the only one done that year, that month, or even that week. You want to know that the team performing your operation is doing plenty of them. This still does not guarantee perfection, but it certainly greatly diminishes the possibility that something will go wrong because of inexperience, a lack of teamwork, or 1 of 100 other reasons.

Good, practical questions to ask are these:

- Is this particular procedure something that's done frequently at this hospital?
- Which group in the city/province/country is doing the highest volume of these procedures?

regional approach. It means, of course, that many patients will have to travel significant distances for this type of care, but the chances of a good outcome are increased substantially.

A very good place to look for data on volumes and outcomes for procedures such as cardiac bypass and complex cancer surgery is the website for the Canadian Institute for Health Information (www.cihi.ca).

2. Know Your Drugs

As discussed in Chapter 5, Canadians now spend more per year on prescription drugs than they do on doctors. Since 1997, the highest spending category after hospitals has been drugs. We take a lot of drugs; they do many of us a great deal of good. Drugs stop infections that might have killed us a generation or two earlier. Drugs allow us to live normal lives despite having many chronic diseases. They ease the pain of arthritis, and they allow asthmatics to breath. But hidden inside this miracle drug world are a few dangerous realities.

Many Canadians are on several drugs at once, and the drugs react and interact with each other in ways that are sometimes dangerous to the health of the patient. Professor Robyn Tamblyn from McGill University has done a great deal of research into the relationship between the accuracy of prescription drugs—that is, the appropriateness of the drug for the medical condition—and the number of doctors and drugs involved. Her findings were that in a patient taking one medication prescribed by one doctor, the odds of accuracy are very high. In other words, 85 to 95 percent of the time this will be the appropriate medication for the condition. However, as the number of doctors involved with a patient's care and the number of prescriptions increase, accuracy declines rapidly. It is not unusual for many Canadian seniors to be taking five or six medications and seeing four or five specialists, in addition to their family doctor. At this point, the chances that all your medications are right, and that they are not interacting with each other in a way hazardous to your health, decline to between 20 and 30 percent. Looked at another way, 70 to 80 percent of the time the situation is less than optimal. A smaller percentage of the time, it is very dangerous. Drug interactions kill thousands of Canadians each year. They make many tens of thousands of Canadians ill when they should be making them well. In addition, one in every nine adult Canadians with health problems reports being given the wrong medication or dose within the past two years.

What can you do about this situation? What if your mother, father, or beloved aunt or uncle is one of those seniors at risk? They are taking a handful of medications each day, trying to keep track of which medications to take before meals and which ones after. So the first important challenge is assisting your loved ones. We presented several good tips on managing medications in

Chapter 10. These tips can be just as successfully applied to non-seniors as well.

As well as understanding the interaction of the medications you are taking, you will need to track your allergies to certain medications. Make sure that everyone who treats you—such as your family doctor, specialists, dentists, and dental surgeons—knows about your allergies.

There are many sources of good information about your medications, but your best resource is actually very close to hand. Canada's pharmacists are well trained in what is now called pharmaceutical care. Their skills go far beyond simply putting the right pills in the right bottle with the right label. They can inform you of possible drug interactions, methods of taking the drugs, and warnings of side effects. You can also consult your pharmacist on over-the-counter medications.

Many of the large pharmacy chains, including Shoppers Drug Mart in its HealthWatch program, will print out a great deal of information about the drug you're taking. The pharmacy's computer system can spot potential drug interactions when you are having a new prescription filled. Following the directions provided when taking your medication is extremely important to get the desired results. Many modern medications need to be taken at exactly the right time, for example. In addition, not all Canadian seniors get all their drugs from the same source. One prescription may be filled at the hospital pharmacy, another filled at Shoppers, another filled somewhere else. You may even be handed some pills on your way out of the hospital. It may be impossible for anyone to fully know all the medications you're on. But you can help by making an effort to fill your prescriptions at a single pharmacy and by keeping a list for your family doctor.

Some provinces have begun to invest in technology to reduce the problem of medications being filled in different places. British Columbia, for example, has an electronic system called Pharmanet that links doctors and pharmacies. An unconscious patient brought into an emergency room in British Columbia will have his or her health card swiped in a card reader. In an instant, the emergency room doctor can know all the medications the patient is taking. Often, from the medications, a doctor can judge what underlying diseases are being treated. For example, a patient on insulin is most certainly to be a diabetic; a patient on Lipitor is likely to have heart disease. Various jurisdictions have invested in technology as a way of reducing medication interactions, but the system is far from perfect. And there are still many occasions when information fails to be available or accurate, to the detriment of patients.

For these reasons, it is important that you take responsibility yourself for knowing what medications you're on. It is also, for a senior you love, well worth having a single pharmacist review all the medications, even if it means putting all the bottles in a plastic bag and going down to the pharmacy. You may find that some shopping centres offer clinics on medications. A pharmacist will root through all your drugs to make sure you are not taking a stale-dated medication, one that is no longer used, or one for which dangerous side effects have been determined. Because of recent spectacular headlines and litigation about deaths resulting from medications such as Celebrex and Vioxx, it is well worth reviewing with your pharmacist or doctor whether you are in a vulnerable category.

Tip

A good source of information about drug dangers and interactions is www.hc-sc.gc.ca. This site links to specific information on drugs that have been recalled or drugs for which warnings have been newly issued by Health Canada. Other good sources of information are disease-specific Internet sites such as those run by the Heart and Stroke Foundation, the Canadian Cancer Society, and the Arthritis Society. Internet addresses for these organizations are listed at the end of Chapter 8.

In a very important recent development, *The British Medical Journal, The New England Journal of Medicine*, and other medical journals are forcing drug companies to make full disclosure of all drug trials—both successful and unsuccessful. They have said they will not publish favourable articles about their drugs unless the companies also post on a freely accessible website the results of trials that failed. This will make public information about when a drug didn't work. This major

Tip

Understand that "medications" includes non-prescription and herbal medications.

breakthrough could allow people to have a far more comprehensive view of the impact of a drug they may be taking or considering taking for their condition.

3. Have the Right Care Team

The third basic step that can improve the safety of your patient care journey is *to know exactly who is giving you care.*

Fortunately, our nation has very well-trained doctors, nurses, pharmacists, and other health professionals. However, not everyone provides quality care. Even the best-trained, qualified provider may fall victim to depression, drug or alcohol addiction, or other situations that compromise the quality of care he or she is delivering. In some cases, colleagues are extremely reluctant to intervene since their relationship may stretch back several decades, through periods in which the doctor or nurse provided excellent care.

The best advice? Be wary! Look out for behaviour or situations that seem odd or inappropriate. It may be something obvious—the doctor's breath smells of alcohol, the doctor makes an inappropriate remark or seems to be acting oddly. Or it may be very subtle—a sense that follow-up care isn't happening when it should.

You need to take action to ensure that the care you're getting is from someone who not only is qualified to give it, by virtue of training, but is delivering it to a high standard. Information is available from regulatory bodies such as colleges of physicians and surgeons on disciplinary actions and complaints against providers who may, for one reason or another, have had previous difficulties providing quality care. You can check whether an individual doctor has been disciplined, sanctioned, or had his or her licence to practise suspended or limited by going to the website of the College of Physicians and Surgeons. Some providers operate under limited licences, which prevents them from doing certain types of procedures.

Tip

Register a complaint with the appropriate agency or regulatory authority. This will help make the system safer. More detail on the art of the complaint is contained in Chapter 14.

4. Know Your Chronic Disease

The average Canadian alive today is likely to live for more than 80 years, which is good news. The inherent problem, however, is that we are not living longer in perfect health. Most Canadians over the age of 70 will find themselves managing one or more chronic diseases.

Right now, some 2.2 million Canadians are living with diabetes, and several million more are living with heart disease, arthritis, and asthma. These conditions have one shared quality: If well managed, they will not prevent people from enjoying fruitful lives. Poorly managed, they have consequences that can be devastating. Poorly managed diabetes can lead to premature blindness and amputation of limbs. Poorly managed asthma can lead to frequent trips to the emergency room in conditions of great distress.

Safe management of chronic disease means understanding your disease in a thorough and thoughtful way. You are likely to have a variety of sources of information. The team treating you will often include more than a physician. For example, diabetics will also be treated by a dietitian and a nurse. If you've been left to manage your diabetes with only occasional visits to a physician, you should consider recruiting a larger team and getting advice from a nurse on issues such as how to care for wounds and pressure sores before they develop into dangerous ulcers; a dietitian can advise you on how you can better manage your diabetes with changes to your diet, a very important aspect of living with diabetes. Seek out information and become an active participant in your own care.

5. Do Not Go Alone

The poet Dylan Thomas wrote, "Do not go gentle into that good night." A modern adaptation would be "Do not go alone or quietly into the health care system." For a safer health care journey, you must have an advocate.

Your advocate can be anyone, a friend, a family member. All that matters is that they care about you. It helps if they are tough-minded. We are not saying health providers don't care about you, but they care about you in what is sometimes an uneven manner. A nurse on one shift might be totally dedicated, qualified, and an extraordinary deliverer of care. A nurse on another shift might be a nervous recent graduate or a burned-out nurse who has done too much overtime and is half asleep on her feet. Often errors happen through combinations of inadvertent events.

Many parts of the health care system have formal, professional patient advocates who handle complaints from individuals. There's nothing wrong with using a professional advocate, but they are often overloaded. A friend or relative who is there to be an advocate can go with you to appointments, monitor the care you receive, ask questions, and essentially do things for you that you would be able to do for yourself if you were well.

When you are alone in a hospital bed, you are at your most vulnerable. A single, simple mistake can cascade into a series of unintended errors. In combination, these mistakes can cause a serious setback to your treatment or bring about a permanent impairment, even death.

A very close friend of Michael's got into enormous trouble following cancer surgery because a meal was brought to her room. Although the surgeon had left very specific instructions that the patient was not to eat, her mother had filled out a meal form when it was brought to her—she presumed the form wouldn't have been brought unless a meal was indicated. The food service staff, following the form, brought the meal to the room, and everyone in the room presumed that since the meal had been delivered, the doctor must have relented and decided it was time for the patient to begin eating again. As a result of consuming a meal before her body was ready for it, the patient's hospital stay was prolonged and she had to endure much additional discomfort. This could have led to quite difficult and permanent consequences. Fortunately in this instance, it didn't, but it underscores the importance of someone double-checking all decisions that affect the patient.

In one hospital in the United States, a whiteboard was hung right over the bed where vital signs were posted, including blood pressure and temperature, so that everyone involved with the case would have the same accurate and timely information. There are many

Questions to Ask in a Hospital

What is the expected recovery time for the patient?
How are the patient's vital signs?
Is the patient ready for a meal?
Is this the right medication?
Is the pain pump that monitors the morphine properly hooked up?
Why is the patient's temperature higher than it was three hours ago?
Why has the patient's medication changed?
Is a fever developing?

methods of getting to quality care, and all of them are based on having full knowledge about the condition of the patient.

The Importance of Accreditation

In 1958, the Canadian hospital accreditation program began. Now the Canadian Council of Health Services Accreditation (www.cchsa.ca) has 400 surveyors who review all types of health organizations in Canada. The surveyors visit hospitals and other health organizations. They apply standards developed in core areas such as Leadership and Partnerships, Human Resources, Information Management, and Environment. Accreditation surveys also compare the performance of health care organizations against standards developed in areas such as cancer care, home care, and acute care. The reports by the accreditors suggest to boards and management teams where there are strengths and where there are weaknesses in the organization. Often the focus is on determining whether the organization has a process in place for safety, for emergency situations, and for ensuring the safety of diagnostic tests. Does the organization measure its own performance? Are the measures robust and consistent? The accreditors also point out areas for improvement.

Most Canadians would be surprised to learn that these accreditation reviews are voluntary in most of Canada. They would also be surprised to learn that the survey results are not generally made public. In 2006, the Health Council of Canada recommended that accreditation be made mandatory for patient safety.

As a patient you should be keenly interested in whether the hospital you are in has been accredited. This assures you, at a minimum, that an external group of experts have examined the organization. You should also be interested in whether a one-, two-, or three-year accreditation award has been granted. In general, the longer the accreditation granted, the better the quality of the health organization. Michael was shocked to learn several years after he left the ministry of health that one Toronto hospital had been granted a meagre six-month accreditation, with recommendations for drastic action. After the report ran on the front page of the *Toronto Star*, the CEO was changed and major improvements set in motion.

Some hospitals and other health organizations make their accreditation reports available to the public. These reports are worth reading. Many Canadians read a movie review or a restaurant review before setting out. Yet often for major or minor surgery involving a hospital stay, we proceed with no advance research. Consider reading the accreditation report of a hospital or health organization review.

RESOURCE GUIDE

ORGANIZATIONS AND ASSOCIATIONS

Canadian Patient Safety Institute
www.patientsafetyinstitute.ca
This site provides information about patient safety efforts in Canada and tips about ensuring your own safety as a patient.

Canadian Institute for Health Information
www.cihi.ca
The CIHI provides broad information on the Canadian health system, including statistics on volumes of operations performed in regions across Canada and their outcomes. It's your best one-stop shop for overall information about Canadian health care services, their quality, and safety.

Longwoods Publishing
www.longwoods.com
Longwoods Publishing, a publisher specializing in health care materials, has provided on the Internet a great deal of information on patient safety.

The National Patient Safety Foundation
www.npsf.org
This organization in the United States has access to a broad array of patient safety information and resources.

The foundation has a bibliography of some 5500 books and articles on patient safety, as well as a speaker's bureau and schedule of upcoming events.

GOVERNMENT PROGRAMS

Health Canada
www.hc-sc.gc.ca
Visit this site for information on drugs and their safety. Health Canada will notify you by e-mail of new developments in the field of adverse drug reaction.

BOOKS

To Err Is Human: Building a Safer Health System, The Institute of Medicine (Washington, D.C.: National Academies Press, 2000).

This landmark American study is available for free online from the Institute of Medicine at National Academies Press, www.nap.edu.

FOURTEEN

Be the Squeaky Wheel—How to Complain Successfully

When the subject of waiting times—or indeed any complaint about the health system—comes up, Michael likes to tell the following story.

> One day I had a call from Lucille, my ex-wife. We are generally on extremely good terms, but on this day Lucille was furious.
>
> "You're always saying this health system works!" I was able to interject, "Not perfectly," before she continued, "Now they're telling me I need a lens implant for my eye, and I'm going to have to wait nine months. How can I possibly do my job if I can't see?"
>
> I offered to help in any way I could. Then I said to her, "Why don't you simply call them back and tell them what you've told me—that it's unacceptable, that you can't wait nine months, that you need

your vision to do your job, your very important job—and see what happens."

She called the hospital back. The response to her forceful presentation of the need for swifter patient care was an appointment to have her eye surgery within a few weeks. She called me back to report her news in a much better mood.

Later that same day, I attended a dinner and encountered the chief executive officer of that same large teaching hospital. He was a good friend and someone I've worked with over the years. I asked him simply, "How do you prioritize your list of patients for eye surgery?" His response, with a smile, was "Squeaky wheel." He went on to elaborate that Canadians are for the most part very patient, and although they may grumble in their beer to their spouses and ex-spouses about the health system, they tend to accept the time frame handed to them. My friend, the hospital CEO, noted that a very small number of people protest when told that they will have a long wait. Often they have a good reason for protesting. In Lucille's case, it was her need to be able to see to do her job.

He further explained, "We call those patients squeaky wheels, and we move them, if not to the top of the line, further toward the top."

You know the old cliché—the squeaky wheel gets the grease. In the health system, the squeaky wheel often gets moved up the queue. People in the health system are human too. They can be persuaded by a cogent argument such as "I need my vision to do my work."

That argument can be considered reasonable if you are behind people who are retired and perhaps need their vision to live but not necessarily to work. Second, the squeaky wheel often gets attention and action simply because we Canadians tend to be very nice people, and our response to someone in distress might well be to try to relieve the distress. In many places in the health system, waiting lists are not terribly well organized or prioritized to begin with. When the waiting list is not prioritized on the basis of any genuine need, the authority to move someone up the queue is likely in the hands of a person at quite a junior level. This is not the case for more major procedures, where a surgeon most likely prioritizes the list based on the needs of the people on it. In that circumstance, you may have far greater difficulty moving up the list if you can't make a compelling argument.

There may come a point in your patient care journey—it may even be early in the journey—when you need to become the squeaky wheel. Let's look at how you go about being heard.

Understanding Your Goal—When to Become Squeaky and How

It is important to understand that any system devised by human beings doesn't always function well or even sensibly. Health care is no exception. You will need to be a forceful advocate on your own behalf or have a forceful advocate working for you. Even with smart navigation and determined advocacy, there may still be occasions when you simply can't get what you need going through the front door. There can be times when becoming the squeaky wheel is the only way you will get the care you need or the redress or financial support you are seeking. To succeed, you need to navigate the myriad complaint routes skilfully. There are many complaints departments and appeal processes in the health system, some of them informal and others formal. They share the attribute that if you do not advocate for your own care, the system will not do it for you.

> **Tip**
>
> Know exactly what you are trying to achieve by complaining. That will help you identify the right avenue for your complaint as well as the tools that will be most effective.

The purpose for the complaint usually falls into one of three broad categories:

1. Complaining or using advocacy to either access care or improve the quality of care you are getting.
2. Complaining to avoid harm to others in the same circumstance. The redress you are seeking is that this same major or minor error or injury not be inflicted on someone else in the future.
3. Complaining for the purpose of gaining compensation to support remedial care or repair when something has gone wrong.

In the first instance, your goal is care; in the second, harm prevention; and in the third, financial redress. Let's go through the reasons for complaining and look at how to best approach them, what your options are, and what tools you can use.

1. Advocating to Improve Your Care or Gain Access

In this first category, you are seeking to influence your patient care journey to take a better direction. Obviously, you are wise to first try to advocate in a positive way. Francesca tells a personal story on page 451 that will illustrate when and how to be tough. Heavy-handed approaches, while at times necessary, should be your final recourse. They should not be your first response.

Whether you have a complaint or not, you should know your rights as a patient. To receive what you are entitled to receive, you first need to understand that you have a right to treatment, a right not to be refused urgent care, a right to a diagnosis, a right to coverage, and even a right to appeal if other rights have not been respected.

Your rights exist at various levels in the health system. At the individual hospital or regional health authority level, there will be a statement of patient rights. Often hospitals will post your rights or make them available in brochure form. This is important information. Once you know what your rights are, it can make advocacy or complaining more focused and effective.

The simplest and most obvious form of advocacy is to refuse to accept what you have been told. You can firmly question decisions conveyed to you and seek redress, such as an earlier appointment. In other cases, particularly where the treatment recommended is major, you may wish to seek a second opinion. Most physicians are open to the idea, but not all. It is essential that you have confidence in both the opinion and the course of treatment. This is not to suggest that there is benefit for "shopping" for an opinion you like. A direct, honest communication with your physician or other provider is the best method. You will not be the first or last patient to seek another opinion. Your family doctor is likely the best source of referral to a second specialist.

For example, a woman facing surgery for breast cancer may seek a second opinion on the merits of lumpectomy, where a small portion of tissue is removed, rather than mastectomy, where the entire breast is removed. For men there are treatments for prostate cancer that involve surgery. There is also watchful waiting, where the condition is monitored but no surgery is performed. The choice may require more than one opinion.

In Chapter 12, "Navigating Canadian Health Care—Swiftly," we dealt primarily with how to harness the support of others. Hospitals have designated people to help advocate on your behalf when things go wrong. One of these is your hospital's patient advocate.

Tip

The Ontario Hospital Association has on its website an excellent document entitled "Your Health Care: Be Involved." It is available in 14 languages at www.oha.com. Choose the Programs bar at the top, Patient Safety and Support Services, then Your Health Care—Be Involved. It will assist your understanding of the in-hospital complaint process.

USING PATIENT ADVOCATES IN HOSPITALS

If you are in a hospital setting and unsatisfied or concerned or in distress, seek out the hospital's patient advocate. As the name implies, the patient advocate is a person employed by the hospital to carry out advocacy on behalf of patients. This work can take the form of intervening on behalf of an individual patient as a kind of caseworker, or it can take the form of making the hospital more patient-centred through broader advocacy.

Don't complain about the hospital food. It is not a strength of hospitals anywhere in the world. The type of complaint that would properly be raised might pertain to pain management or its absence, poor communication by a nurse, or concern about fever or other symptoms. The patient advocate is your first resort after a simple concern expressed to the staff caring for you.

When you are in hospital, your doctor can be your most important and knowledgeable advocate. Enlist his or her support in solving any problems you are having with care. If your complaint is about the doctor, you should seek redress from the department head or from the patient advocate's office. If those avenues fail to secure action, you may need to take a more formal route by contacting the vice president responsible for patient care or the president of the hospital. You may simply be referred to the patient advocate.

BEING AN ADVOCATE FOR YOURSELF OR YOUR LOVED ONE

The Ontario Psychiatric Patient Advocate Office (www.ppao.gov.on.ca) provides a four-step program on self-advocacy that has application beyond mental health services. It is a straightforward approach that involves a few basic principles:

1. Define the problem so that you can communicate it clearly and in an understandable fashion. You need to ensure that your explanation of events or issues is not so complicated and lengthy that busy caregivers tune you out. Sometimes defining the problem succinctly is trickier than it seems. It can be tougher to write a short essay than a long one because in a long essay you can talk about everything. In a short one you have to know all the points and include only those that are the most important.
2. Develop your action plan. You may want to consider options that you have available. This will help you set realistic goals that improve your chances of success. You will need to know who to

approach and what information to approach them with to make a compelling case. It is very important that you contact the most appropriate person at the beginning. The Ontario Psychiatric Patient Advocate Office suggests that you first go to the decision-maker closest to the issue and work your way up through the various levels of decision-making. Don't escalate your issue too soon. You may end up getting noses out of joint when you don't have to. Also, you should ensure that you are clear about what your goal is. This is key throughout the entire process.

3. Put your plan into action. This involves presenting your complaint and getting people to listen to you. It is important that you also listen to others and be ready to negotiate with them to resolve your problem. Be aware of how you communicate in situations such as these. You may be someone who quickly becomes angry or emotional, or perhaps you're someone who runs out of steam easily. Try to remain calm, open-minded, and flexible, but be firm if you feel you are still being misunderstood or brushed off.
4. Evaluate the results. Think about what you have accomplished and how. What would you have done differently and why? Even if you are less than satisfied, you have taken the important step of voicing your concern. This will help you in your next patient journey.

Tips

When you are entering a hospital, get the phone number and office location of the patient advocate.

Make your case for better care by clearly sharing your concerns with your care providers. They typically want to help, if you let them in to your world. People who are treated kindly will often respond in kind.

If you are going to make a complaint, be sure you have all the documentation you need. This would include a detailed account of events, any test results, medical records, and other material that would support your complaint.

Make sure you have recorded the names of persons with whom you spoke and the date.

Be clear about the next steps in the complaint process and who is responsible for doing specific tasks.

Make sure you take your issue to someone at a higher level of authority if you need to. Also, make sure that it is the right person, and that you don't escalate things too soon.

This approach is well worth considering when you are not getting care or when the quality of that care is not meeting your expectations. Having a plan is an excellent way of clarifying what is realistic and how to get it.

2. Complaining to Prevent Harm to Others

If you have gone through a negative experience but there is nothing that can be done to help you specifically, you may find it worthwhile registering a complaint to prevent similar situations from happening to others. As individuals, we have access to a range of regulatory bodies, including colleges of physicians and surgeons and colleges of nurses.

Provincial governments create colleges to regulate different types of health providers. For example, Ontario regulates midwives, pharmacists, optometrists, chiropractors, dentists, and other health disciplines—a total of 23 regulated health professions under 21 regulatory colleges. These colleges are generally self-governing, but they have some public representation from citizen governors. Beyond the complaints at the regulatory level there is a resort to the courts (see "Complaining to Get Redress or Compensation").

This next story is a great example of the importance of knowing your rights, and of knowing when and how to be the squeaky wheel. It incorporates two categories of advocacy and complaints described above: advocating for better care and complaining to prevent harm to others. It shows when you need to get tough, and how and when to escalate pressure in a reasonable manner.

This is Francesca's story:

> By and large, I do believe that making allies in the health system is the best approach to getting better care. But sometimes, when that doesn't work, you need to get tough to get the care you need. And if mistakes were made along the way, you need to file a complaint to help ensure that these mistakes do not happen to someone else. I believe that is not only your right but your duty.

One day my husband, Steve, started feeling terribly sharp abdominal pains that would leave him doubled over. Over the course of the next two weeks, he was visited at home by two different doctors (his family doctor was on holidays). The first told him it was a viral infection; the second told him it was a bacterial infection and put him on antibiotics. Neither of the two doctors considered appendicitis, since the pain was not in the area of the appendix. Neither doctor ran a single test, even though Steve had none of the symptoms that is associated with infection (viral or otherwise). He did not get better, and he kept experiencing these pains in spite of the treatment.

Three days later, we were on the way to our cottage when Steve doubled over with severe pain again. My father had always told me that with antibiotics, you usually start to feel a difference within 48 hours, but Steve was now into 72 hours. I called my father, who was adamant that we turn the car around and go to a full-service hospital with a good emergency department.

"This guy needs tests!" my father bellowed into the phone. My dad was convinced that this pain could be appendicitis, even if it was not in the right location. He was shocked that no one had bothered to take a single test, even though Steve didn't have any of the other symptoms that one would associate with an intestinal infection, such as fever or diarrhea.

So on a holiday weekend, we turned the car back and drove to a Toronto hospital. Once there, the hospital ran X-rays and blood tests, which revealed nothing. The hospital staff informed us that there was only one test left to do, an ultrasound. Unfortunately, the ultrasound technician was at home and was to be called only in case of an emergency. The hospital wanted Steve out. They told us that he could return Monday for the test.

Once again, I called my father, whose instructions were clear: "You do not leave the hospital without a diagnosis. The ultrasound needs to be done. I am convinced he has appendicitis, and this is very serious. An appendix can burst and turn into a peritonitis, which can kill you. Furthermore, once it's burst, there is a very narrow window in which to operate. . . . Do *not* leave the hospital without a diagnosis!"

The health care system was failing us. I thought of the comedy of errors that we had already been through:

1. The first doctor didn't investigate.
2. The second prescribed medicine but didn't investigate.
3. The hospital was pushing for discharge even though they knew there was still a test that needed to be done and there was still no diagnosis.

It was then that I saw first-hand how difficult it is to be an advocate. The emergency room was packed. Trauma cases were coming in from everywhere. No one wanted to listen to me. I thought hard about a game plan. My job was to keep him in the hospital and get that ultrasound! That was my goal! I had pleaded and tried to get the staff to call the technician. They would not.

Just then I glanced at a bulletin board. On a brochure I saw the words "Patients' Rights." Under the heading, in smaller print, I began to read: "You have the right to be treated in the hospital. You have the right to a diagnosis." Aha! There it was!

Know your rights! I could have, and should have, asked earlier for the hospital's patient rights policy. Luckily, I didn't have to.

I took the paper off the board and marched up to the head nurse (who by now wanted to shoot me). I showed her the pamphlet. "There is no diagnosis and one more test needs to be done. I am sorry, but we simply won't leave until that happens." I was angry and adamant.

Frustrated, she called the ultrasound technician. He arrived, and within a few minutes, we received word that Steve had a burst appendix and the toxins were making their way through his system. The fever began shortly after—soon he would be too unstable to operate on. The flurry that ensued was impressive. Steve was operated on and, after a five-month ordeal, was well again.

It may have been over for him, but not for me. I realized that I had a responsibility to ensure this didn't happen again. My father had often told me that diagnosis of an appendix can be tricky. Tests don't always reveal that there is a problem until it is dire. So what did I have to complain about?

Simple: The two doctors who visited Steve didn't *try* to investigate. I am not a doctor, but when someone drops to the ground, doubled over with pain repeatedly for days, I think that person might be in trouble. And the fact that a test may fail to

> reveal the problem is no excuse to do no investigation at all.
>
> I called the College of Physicians and Surgeons of Ontario. I told them upfront that I was not interested in launching a lawsuit. My interest was to record a complaint to ensure that these two doctors were informed about the outcome of Steve's case. If a doctor gets a call from the college on a performance issue, I hope he will handle the next case differently.
>
> You can't take issue with a doctor for not finding the problem. I believe you can take issue with a doctor for not trying. With regard to the hospital, I did enough complaining that no further grief was necessary. My point had been made. A serious error had been averted.

As noted above, your avenue of complaint is to the appropriate college. After consideration of the complaint, including correspondence with the doctor or nurse, the college will decide whether the situation warrants a fuller investigation and hearing. Those who have complaints lodged against them are informed of the complaint according to the procedures established by the college. In a serious case, there is a formal hearing, and discipline, up to and including loss of licence, can occur.

3. Complaining to Get Redress or Compensation

In Canada, we are not nearly as litigious as Americans, but there is a continuing resort to the courts by people who believe they were injured in some fashion by a stay in the hospital, a surgical procedure, or a misdiagnosis of some condition or illness. There are lawyers who specialize in medical malpractice, but you should know that litigation is a lengthy and difficult process.

If you believe you are being damaged by your treatment or are not getting the treatment you should, the first question you must ask yourself is whether you can gain access to someone with the authority to improve the care you are receiving. You must do that rapidly. If you are injured, the most important thing is to have the injury redressed rapidly, rather than engaging in a long process of litigation to pursue compensation. The issue of payment is a separate one. For example, the government may decide that a certain new procedure is not yet an "insured service" under provincial legislation. If you require a new and very expensive cancer drug that has not yet been approved by the provincial government, their refusal may, because of the enormous cost, prevent your access. Your first avenue is to appeal to the relevant board. Beyond that, the courts are your forum of appeal. But in the short term, the media may be your best recourse, particularly if the drug is life extending.

In some cases, where the damage is already done, legal redress to receive financial compensation may be the only available route.

The most expensive malpractice cases usually involve birthing errors. This is because, to redress the damage, courts award settlements that provide for lifelong care for the damaged infant. In a Canadian birth case, a family was eventually awarded $3.3 million by the courts. This award was made to the family of an eight-year-old child who contracted herpes simplex shortly after she was born in 1993. The herpes virus caused serious, permanent disabilities, rendering the child a quadriplegic with impairment to hearing, sight, and brain function.

The cause came to light only because the child's grandmother read an article in *Reader's Digest* and contacted the world-renowned herpes simplex expert Dr. Stephen Sacks. It was his testimony, and the testimony of other experts, that convinced the court that if the doctor had used a widely accepted treatment for newborns with herpes symptoms, the damage would have been prevented.

The total settlement was $200,000 in damages, $1.5 million for future care, $167,000 for care provided by her mother and grandmother since birth, and a further $1.5 million for medical equipment and a specially built house.

If you will have ongoing expenses for someone injured as a result of poor medical care, you have recourse to the courts and are best advised to seek competent legal counsel. Many of these cases, such as the one above, concern the care of a baby injured during the birthing process. Not all birthing injuries are the result of malpractice, however. Birthing is a normally safe process, but errors, lack of knowledge, or the lack of application of a widely accepted treatment can result in horrific injuries.

Navigating the legal system is a topic that could fill a separate book, and we are not qualified to write that book. But you should know that pursuing redress via the system is a long, arduous, and complicated process, and you are best advised by a specialist in medical malpractice. Many of the large law firms in Canada have such specialists, and they are the ones to consult about the merits of your case.

Physicians in Canada belong to the Canadian Medical Protective Association (CMPA), a large insurer that will defend physicians in a lawsuit. Hospitals similarly carry insurance. Although occasionally you read of a patient receiving a large settlement, many, many cases are not pursued because of the costs to the parties involved.

The CMPA charges premiums to doctors, and in some provinces the premiums are heavily subsidized by payments from provincial governments, a policy that was negotiated by physicians' bargaining agents. The CMPA views this as part of the doctors' compensation, not a government subsidy. It is both—in truth, a negotiated subsidy. As a consequence, the CMPA has a fund of $1 billion to spend on behalf of physicians in legal malpractice suits. It is not surprising, then, that a patient will not embark lightly on a journey down the legal avenue. But if you are faced with compelling evidence of malpractice resulting in horrific damage, you may have little choice.

Tip

If you are even remotely considering litigation, be careful to keep all documents and to make detailed notes of what you were told and what you or your loved one experienced. Note the names of nurses and others involved with the case. All of this fact-gathering will be valuable to a lawyer advising whether your case has merit. Often, medical legal cases turn on the credibility of witnesses and evidence. As non-physicians, most patients start at a disadvantage in court. The best way of levelling the playing field is to have detailed documentation.

Another type of case is illustrated by the example of a hepatitis B class-action suit. Of thousands of patients who received treatment at one of the clinics run by Dr. Ronald Wilson in southern Ontario, about a thousand were infected with hepatitis B when a technologist, Nicolas Kyprianou, did not wear protective gloves and did not use properly sterilized needles during routine electroencephalogram procedures. These infected patients undertook a class-action lawsuit, which they won in what up to that time (2002) was the largest settlement for medical malpractice in Canada.

Class-action lawsuits are becoming more common in Canada. If you're part of a group of people who have been injured, you can band together in a single lawsuit. The advantage of the class-action lawsuit is that generally the cost is borne by all the defendants, thus making it more affordable for each individual. Lawyers are more likely to take on a class-action suit because of the number of plaintiffs. Usually in these cases, the lawyers' compensation is a percentage of the final judgment. The lawyers bear the cost and risk of pursuing the litigation, rather than the plaintiffs. In successful suits the lawyers gain a portion of the settlement.

Recent class-action suits in Canada have been brought by those injured by tainted blood and by women in Quebec receiving delayed radiation therapy after surgery for breast cancer.

Tactics

In all three of these categories of advocacy and/or complaints, there are tactics that can be used to move your case forward.

1. Political Recourse

This tactic can be used at any time but is most effective in the first category—when you are trying to get better care. Beyond the formal appeals within the health system, you can make direct appeals to the political level—to the member who represents you in your provincial or territorial legislature, the member who represents you in the federal Parliament, or the office of the provincial ministry of health. Each of these elected officials has staff dedicated to individual casework. These people possess the knowledge and contacts to be helpful in many instances. The office of the chair of your regional health facility or hospital board is another place to seek assistance. As we said earlier, many hospitals and health organizations can be very useful in this effort, as they have formal patient advocates. Your goal is to try to drum up support from political people to help run interference with the health care system. Often patient advocates will call a minister's office to request help in a difficult situation. Sometimes this move is very effective.

2. The Media

Getting the media on board with your story can be effective when you need to complain. At a national level, there are a handful of superstars in the health-reporting world. One of Canada's best investigative journalists is Lisa Priest. In 1998, she wrote *Operating in the Dark*, an insightful examination of safety problems in Canadian health care. Recently Priest, who now writes for *The Globe and Mail* newspaper, received a Michener Award in Journalism for work she had done to improve cancer care. Another journalist who also writes for *The Globe and Mail* is André Picard, who did extraordinary work on the tainted blood tragedy and its victims. Finally, *Globe* columnist Margaret Wente covers a far broader beat than health care, but she writes with power and passion and has included health issues in the topics she comments on.

At the CBC, Wendy Mesley has a show—*Marketplace*—that goes to bat for those without power. Mesley, as a cancer patient, produced a tough-minded documentary asking important questions about cancer.

At a local level, you can readily identify the health reporter by scanning the pages of your local newspaper.

You can also call the newsroom and ask who covers health stories.

Seeking out a journalist with your story can be effective, but it should not be your first course of action. It can allow you leverage, however, particularly if your case is one of a group of cases. It is important to remember that access to the media is hit and miss. Not all stories make the front page.

> **Tip**
>
> If you can get an introduction to a journalist through a mutual acquaintance who can vouch for your credibility, do it. Be clear and balanced with the journalist. She is looking for a story, not your tirade or frustration. Let her hear your story and take it from there.

3. Regulatory Colleges and Hospital Quality Committees

Canadian health professionals—doctors, nurses, pharmacists, and others—are governed by regulatory bodies in each province. In general, these bodies issue licences to practitioners and review any complaints. For example, physicians and surgeons are licensed and occasionally disciplined by the provincial college of physicians and surgeons.

All postgraduate residents and all practising physicians must hold an educational or practice licence from the medical regulatory authority in the province in which they study or practice.

Patients with concerns can lodge complaints with their provincial colleges. They can also contact the hospital's quality committee. In both cases, your best outcome would be action to prevent others from having experiences similar to your own. If the problem you experienced occurred in a hospital, the quality committee would be a logical forum after hospital management. If the adverse outcome did not result from a hospital stay, the regulatory college may be your only option, short of the courts. It is best to proceed with the hospital quality committee prior to contacting the regulatory college, rather than the other way around. Once you have complained to a college, others may stand aside, given the formal nature of the college procedures.

COLLEGES

When you launch a complaint with a regulatory college, there is certain information you will need to provide and processes you will go through. Here is the complaints process at the College of Physicians and Surgeons of Ontario:

1. You send in your complaint in writing, on tape, on film, or on disc. Your complaint can be sent by e-mail, but the college will reply by regular mail for confidentiality purposes.
2. An investigator from the college will contact you by phone or letter. Your concerns can be clarified

at this point, and you can provide additional information. Your concerns may even be resolved through this initial contact.

3. If the complaint is to proceed, the college notifies the doctor by phone or letter. By law, the doctor must be provided with details about the complaint and must be allowed to respond.
4. The college must be given authority to have access to the relevant medical information. The person who has authority to allow a patient's medical information to be released is the one who gives consent. That could be you, if it's your own medical information, or you acting as power of attorney for someone else. This information can be gathered from the doctor about whom you are complaining, as well as from other doctors or health care professionals and facilities.
5. If a resolution has not yet been reached, the college asks the doctor to respond to the complaint. The doctor then has an opportunity to explain the care or conduct that is at issue.
6. At this point, the college will ask for the medical information about your case to be released so a complete investigation can be undertaken.
7. The college investigator prepares the materials so they can be reviewed by the complaints committee, which is made up of six doctors and three members of the public. Both the doctor and the complainant are notified of the date of the

meeting, but neither meets with the committee. The committee may make its decision based on this information, or it may decide more information is needed. If the committee decides that the complaint has no merit (it is frivolous, was made in bad faith, or is an abuse of process, for example) it will not investigate further, but this is a rare occurrence.

8. The committee may find that the doctor provided appropriate care or that no misconduct occurred; it may caution the doctor in writing if the committee believes this to be appropriate; ask the doctor to appear before the committee for a caution, with advice on how to avoid the problem in future; direct the doctor to the quality assurance committee, where he or she may be asked to take part in educational programs; direct the doctor to the college's executive committee (if the complaints committee has concerns about the doctor's health that will affect his or her ability to practise); send concerns about the doctor to the discipline committee; or decide not to investigate further because the complaint is without merit.
9. Both the doctor and the complainant are given a copy of the decision, usually within two months of the meeting.
10. Both the doctor and the complainant can appeal the finding.

Your main expectation of a college process should be to record your complaint. It is possible that the physician, nurse, or other health professional will be censured in some fashion. Every year a few practitioners lose their licence to practise, usually for extreme conduct and often for a finite period of time. Still others have their licence limited. They must practise with supervision or are barred from performing certain types of work.

Some of these colleges are listed in the Resources section at the end of this chapter.

HOSPITAL QUALITY COMMITTEES

Hospitals have quality committees at the board level. The purpose of the quality committee is to improve the quality of care provided and to mitigate the hospital's risks. These committees are at the governance level and are generally made up of leading citizens. For example, former premier of Ontario Bob Rae chaired Toronto's University Health Network quality committee for a time. A letter to the chair of this committee, copied to the CEO and others, may yield an investigation. Your letter should detail your complaint with as much clarity and evidence as possible. You should also list those in a position to support your point of view. It is best not to include threats of legal action, as that may cause the committee to hand your letter off to the hospital's lawyers without considering its merits.

4. Formal Appeal Boards

You have a right to appeal if you are refused public paid coverage for treatment. However, your right varies significantly from province to province. Even within one province's legislation there are a range of appeal provisions. For example, the Ontario Health Services Appeal and Review Board (www.hsarb.on.ca), an independent quasi-judicial tribunal, has a review and appeal mandate under 14 different statutes, ranging from the Health Insurance Act to the Immunization of School Pupils Act. The website sets out the rules for an appeal as well as answers to frequent questions.

Each province has a formal appeals board that deals with cases when, for example, you are denied coverage for a procedure by your jurisdiction's medicare plan; this happens when a particular procedure is viewed as experimental. If you are denied coverage, you are entitled to an appeal. This appeal goes to a formal board, which generally consults external medical experts on the question of whether the procedure is routine and simply not available in Ontario or Saskatchewan, or wherever it is you are, or whether it is regarded as experimental. Having a physician advocating on your behalf can be very important to winning at this stage. It is also important to research precedents so that you know whether the appeal mechanism has in fact proven some other cases in the past. You have the option of being represented by a lawyer, but it is not a requirement. The cost of a lawyer needs to be weighed against the potential benefit of a successful appeal. If you are undertaking an appeal over tens of thousands of disputed payment dollars, a lawyer may be a wise investment. If your appeal is over a few hundred dollars and the principle of it, then a lawyer may be a costly vanity.

Tip

Start with internal complaints. If you are not satisfied, move your appeal to the management and political level. If that does not work, take your case to the media. If that fails, consult a lawyer.

Reaching Safe Harbour

Our recurring theme in this book has been that you will get a better and faster outcome from the Canadian health care system—you will reach your safe harbour—if you become a skilled, knowledgeable navigator. As we wrote this book, patient advocates in the United States were successful in persuading the Bush administration to approve a bill passing into law the Patient Navigator, Outreach and Chronic Disease Prevention Act. This act puts $25 million into a demonstration program for patient navigation and outreach. Grants will be given to support the recruitment, training, and employment of patient navigators. These patient navigators will have six duties:

1. Coordinating health care services and provider referrals

2. Facilitating the involvement of community organizations that can help with access to services
3. Notifying patients of, and facilitating enrolment in, clinical trials
4. Assisting patients in overcoming barriers within the health care system to ensure prompt diagnosis and treatment
5. Coordinating with the health insurance ombudsman to help patients covered by public programs or private insurance
6. Conducting ongoing outreach to disparate health communities—that is, communities that do not have good access to health care, such as areas of poverty and immigrant communities

Even though Canadian health care is becoming more complex, it is a simple system compared to that in the United States. As a result of great numbers of competing insurers and insurance plans, Americans absolutely need professional navigators. This program is a three-year experiment that we hope will demonstrate what the approach can actually achieve for patients.

As long as Canada does not have professional patient navigators in our health care system, however, it is up to each of us, working with medical professionals, to chart and sail our own course.

RESOURCE GUIDE

PATIENT ADVOCACY

While not directly relevant to gaining redress in Canada, the National Patient Advocate Foundation in Washington, D.C., provides a rich array of policy, legislative, and research initiatives on the topic of patient safety. Access the foundation's website at www.npaf.org.

COMPLAINT AND APPEAL MECHANISMS

You may need to search carefully on these websites to find information about the complaint process.

College of Physicians and Surgeons of British Columbia
www.cpsbc.ca
E-mail: questions@cpsbc.ca or registration@cpsbc.ca
Telephone: (604) 733-7758 or 1-800-461-3008
Fax: (604) 733-3503 (general); (604) 694-6104 (registration)
858 Beatty Street, Suite 400
Vancouver, BC V6B 1C1

College of Physicians and Surgeons of Alberta
www.cpsa.ab.ca
Telephone: (780) 423-4764 or 1-800-561-3899 (public inquiries)
Fax: (780) 420-0651
900 Manulife Place

10180—101 Street
Edmonton, AB T5J 4P8

College of Physicians and Surgeons of Saskatchewan
www.quadrant.net/cpss
E-mail: cpss@quadrant.net
Telephone: (306) 244-7355 or 1-800-667-1668
Fax: (306) 244-0090 (general); (306) 244-2600 (registrar)
321A 21st Street East, Suite 500
Saskatoon, SK S7K 0C1

College of Physicians and Surgeons of Manitoba
www.cpsm.mb.ca
Telephone: (204) 774-4344
Fax: (204) 774-0750
1000–1661 Portage Avenue
Winnipeg, MB R3J 3T7

College of Physicians and Surgeons of Ontario
www.cpso.on.ca
E-mail: feedback@cpso.on.ca
Telephone: (416) 967-2603 or 1-800-268-7096 (general)
80 College Street
Toronto, ON M5G 2E2

Collège des médecins du Québec
www.cmq.org
E-mail: info@cmq.org

Telephone: (514) 933-4441 or 1-888-MÉDECIN
Fax: (514) 933-3112
2170 boulevard René-Lévesque Ouest
Montreal, QC H3H 2T8

College of Physicians and Surgeons of New Brunswick
www.cpsnb.org
E-mail: info@cpsnb.org
Telephone: (506) 849-5050 or 1-800-667-4641
Fax: (506) 849-5069
1 Hampton Road, Suite 300
Rothesay, NB E2E 5K8

College of Physicians and Surgeons of Nova Scotia
www.cpsns.ns.ca
Telephone: (902) 422-5823 or 1-877-282-7767 (toll-free)
Fax: (902) 422-5035
Sentry Place, Suite 200
1559 Brunswick Street
Halifax, NS B3J 2G1

College of Physicians and Surgeons of Prince Edward Island
www.cpspei.ca
Telephone: (902) 566-3861
Fax: (902) 566-3861
199 Grafton Street, Suite 401
Charlottetown, PE C1A 1L2

College of Physicians and Surgeons of Newfoundland and Labrador
www.nmb.ca
E-mail: nmb@thezone.net
Telephone: (709) 726-8546
Fax: (709) 726-4725
139 Water Street, Suite 603
St. John's, NL A1C 1B2

Yukon Medical Council
www.community.gov.yk.ca
E-mail: ymc@gov.yk.ca
Telephone: (867) 667-5257
Fax: (867) 667-3609
c/o Registrar of Medical Practitioners
P.O. Box 2703 C-5
Whitehorse, YT Y1A 2C6

Northwest Territories Health and Social Services
www.hlthss.gov.nt.ca/english/services/health_care_service
_complaints/default.htm
E-mail: professional_licensing@gov.nt.ca
Telephone: (867) 920-8058
Fax: (867) 873-0484
Government of the Northwest Territories
P.O. Box 1320
Yellowknife, NT X1A 2L9

Nunavut Department of Health and Social Services
www.gov.nu.ca
Telephone: (867) 975-5700
Fax: (867) 975-5705
Government of Nunavut
Registrar, Professional Licensing
NCC Building, 2nd Floor
P.O. Box 390
Kugluktuk, NU X0B 0E0

The Royal College of Physicians and Surgeons of Canada is the national body that oversees examinations of physicians and surgeons.
The Royal College of Physicians and Surgeons of Canada
www.rcpsc.medical.org
Telephone: (613) 730-8177 or 1-800-668-3740 (toll-free)
774 Echo Drive
Ottawa, ON K1S 5N8

MEDIA

Every city in Canada has newspapers, radio stations, and television stations. Even small towns usually have a daily or weekly newspaper. All have reporters who need stories to fill their pages or air time. It would require a lengthy tome to set out all the contact information, but you should have no difficulty finding news outlets. Look for a sympathetic reporter to whom you can tell your story.

Two websites can connect you to hundreds of media outlets:

www.kidon.com
Kidon claims to link you to 872 individual media outlets.

www.mondotimes.com
Mondo Times also provides many links.

LEGAL CONTACTS

Get in touch with your provincial bar association to seek out its medical law section. A web search of lawyers in your community is another route.

www.lawmedmal.ca
This site lists by city dozens of Canadian law firms that have specialists in medical malpractice.

Afterword

In *Navigating Canada's Health Care* we have shared our stories, insights, and tips to promote more successful patient journeys. We hope to have aided some of our readers in finding their way more swiftly and safely through the complexities of Canadian health care.

We believe that Canadians need to be more proactive when it comes to our health care. We need to be able to share experiences, lessons learned, tips, and resources. We need to be informed consumers and citizens and better understand what is making the news in health care and how it affects the way it is delivered in our province, territory, or country.

Our hope is to write a sequel to *Navigating* using some of the patient stories posted on our website. What we will be looking for are stories that provide lessons or tips that others might benefit from. We are sympathetic if you had only a negative experience, but unless it yields useful advice, we would prefer to focus on insights and lessons in how to navigate more successfully. Please let us know at the end of your story whether you are willing to allow us to share it with others.

Our website address is www.navigatingcanadashealth-care.ca (type in the name of the book with no apostrophe or spaces).

Thank you in advance for your assistance.

Michael B. Decter
Francesca Grosso
2006

Government Resource Guide

This guide is intended to supplement the Resources sections at the end of each chapter.

Government of Canada

Navigate to the right provincial or territorial program or office using www.canadabenefits.gc.ca. This website is well organized and will get you the provincial or territorial contact information that you seek on any topic. It is easy to navigate. You will see two columns. The first is labelled "I Am." Click on who you are—a parent, a senior, a student, etc. The second column is entitled "Life Events." Click on the issue for which you need to contact your government—for example, "Health Concerns." Click on the province or territory that interests you and all the provincial and territorial programs will be listed, with complete contact information and links.

Provincial and Territorial Health Ministries

Here is a list of resources that should be your first point of contact for information about assistive device programs, home care, or funded nursing homes in your province or territory.

ALBERTA

From within the Province of Alberta (all numbers are toll-free):

- Alberta Health Care, dial 310-0000, then dial (780) 427-1432
- Health and Wellness Ministry Information, dial 310-0000, then dial (780) 427-7164
- Aids to Daily Living, dial 310-0000, then dial (780) 427-0731

From outside Alberta, call:

- Alberta Health Care, (780) 427-1432
- Health and Wellness General Information, (780) 427-7164
- Provincial Government General Information, (780) 427-2711

Deaf/hearing-impaired callers, dial:

- (780) 427-9999 in Edmonton to reach the provincial government
- 1-800-232-7215 from elsewhere in Alberta to reach the provincial government

BRITISH COLUMBIA

Ministry of Health Services, Health Information Line: 1-800-465-4911 (toll-free); (250) 952-1742

Ministry of Human Resources, Enhanced Medical Coverage

Health Benefits Branch: 1-888-221-7711 (toll-free)

Disability Benefits: 1-800-337-3531 (toll-free)

MANITOBA

Manitoba Health Office: 1-800-392-1207 (toll-free)

TDD/TTY: (204) 774-8618

Home Care Equipment Program: (204) 945-8611

www.gov.mb.ca

To find regional health authorities on this website, scroll down to "Health" and then click on "Regional Health Authorities." You can contact the local health authority, which will ultimately be responsible for any needs assessments for both home care and funded nursing homes. If you scroll to "Health" and click on "Info Health Guide," you will get information about general provincial policy on a variety of topics, with links to the organizations you will need to contact.

NEW BRUNSWICK

Department of Family and Community Services: (506) 453-2001

NEWFOUNDLAND AND LABRADOR

Health and Community Services: (709) 729-4984

NORTHWEST TERRITORIES

Department of Health and Social Services, Health Benefits Programs: 1-800-661-0830 (toll-free); (867) 777-7400

NOVA SCOTIA

Department of Health: 1-800-387-6665 (toll-free); (902) 424-5818; TDD/TTY: 1-800-670-8888 (toll-free)

NUNAVUT

Department of Health and Social Services: (867) 975-5700

ONTARIO

1-800-268-1154 (toll-free); (416) 314-5518
TDD/TTY: 1-800-387-5559 (toll-free);
(416) 327-4282
Assistive Devices and Home Oxygen Program:
1-800-268-6021 (toll-free); (416) 327-8804
www.health.gov.on.ca
To find Community Care Access Centres from this website, click on "Home, Community and Residential

Care Services for Seniors," then on "Find a Community Care Access Centre."

PRINCE EDWARD ISLAND

Department of Health: (902) 368-4900

QUEBEC

Ministry of Health and Social Services: 1-800-707-3380 (toll-free)
Health Insurance Plan: 1-800-561-9749 (toll-free)
Quebec: (418) 646-4636; Montreal: (514) 864-3411
Handicapped Services: 1-800-567-1465 (toll-free); (819) 475-8585
TDD/TTY: 1-800-567-1477 (toll-free)

SASKATCHEWAN

Health Registration Branch: 1-800-667-7551 (toll-free); (306) 787-3475
Aids to Independent Living Program: (306) 787-7121

YUKON

Department of Health and Social Services: 1-800-661-0408 (toll-free); (867) 667-5209
Pharmacare and Extended Health Care Benefits Program: (867) 667-2403

Notes

CHAPTER 1

page 4 **"The CIHI also tells us that"**: Canadian Institute for Health Information, *Giving Birth in Canada: A Regional Health Profile*. Ottawa: Canadian Institute for Health Information, 2004.

page 21 **"According to some research, women who work with a doula"**: E. D. Hodnett, S. Gates, G. J. Hofmeyr, and C. Sakala, "Continuous Support for Women During Childbirth, *The Cochrane Library*, Issue 3, 2006. John Wiley & Sons, Ltd.

page 34 **"CIHI reports that most jurisdictions"**: Canadian Institute for Health Information, *Giving Birth in Canada: The Costs*. Ottawa: Canadian Institute for Health Information, 2006.

CHAPTER 2

page 52 **"The importance of experience is made clear"**: A. Guttmann, D. Manuel, P. Dick, T. To, K. Lam, and T. Stukel, "Volume Matters: Physician Practice Characteristics and Immunization Coverage in Young Children Insured Through a Universal Health Plan," *Pediatrics* 117 (3), 2000: 595–602.

page 69 **"Teenagers and young adults"**: Statistics Canada, *Canadian Community Health Survey: Mental Health and Well-Being*. Ottawa, 2003.

page 70 **"According to an article"**: C. Waddell, D. Offord, C. A. Shepherd, J. M. Hua, and K. McEwan, "Child Psychiatric Epidemiology and Canadian Public Policy-making: The State of the Science and the Art of the Possible," *Canadian Journal of Psychiatry* 47 (9), 2002: 825–32.

page 70 **"In its *Report on Mental Illnesses*"**: Health Canada, A Report on Mental Illnesses in Canada. Health Canada: Ottawa: Health Canada, 2002.

page 76 **"A link between body weight"**: L. Oliver and M. Hayes, "Neighbourhood Socioeconomic Status and the Prevalence of Overweight Canadian Children and Youth," *Canadian Journal of Public Health* 96 (6), 2005: 415–20.

CHAPTER 5

page 142 **"Prescription drugs cost the Canadian"**: *Canadian CompuScript Audit* published by IMS Health Canada, 2006.

page 142 **"It is staggering"**: Canadian Institute for Health Information, *Health Care in Canada 2005*. Ottawa: CIHI, 2005.

page 148 **"Overall, government plans spend"**: Canadian Institute for Health Information, *Health Care in Canada 2005*. Ottawa: CIHI, 2005.

page 149 **"An article by Wendy Ungar"**: Wendy Ungar and Maciej Witkos, "Public Drug Plan Coverage for Children Across Canada: A Portrait of Too Many Colours," *Healthcare Policy* 1 (1):100–122, 2005.

page 152 **"The Canadian Institute for Health information reported"**: Canadian Institute for Health Information, *Explaining the 70/30 Split: How Canada's Health Care System Is Financed*, 2005.

CHAPTER 8

page 252 **"'The world is experiencing a rapid rise'"**: World Health Organization, *Preparing a Health Care*

Workforce for the 21st Century: The Challenge of Chronic Conditions, World Health Organization, Geneva, Switzerland, 2005, p. 15.

page 262 **"'Canada has a diabetes epidemic.'"**: Canadian Diabetic Association and Diabète Québec, *Diabetes Report*, 2005.

page 263 **"For example, a study has shown"**: Stewart Harris, J. M. Eokoe, Y. Zdanowicz, and S. Webster-Bogaert, "Glycemic Control and Morbidity in the Canadian Primary Care Setting (Results of the Diabetes in Canada Evaluation Study)," *Diabetes Research and Clinical Practice*, October 2005, pp. 90–97.

CHAPTER 10

page 315 **"In 2003, people over 65"**: Canadian Institute for Health Information, *Health Care in Canada 2003.* Ottawa: CIHI, 2003.

CHAPTER 12

page 392 **"The Canadian Institute for Health Information recently"**: Canadian Institute for Health Information, *Understanding Emergency Department Wait Times*, 2005.

page 403 **"Another aspect of this paper-based system"**: Canada Health Infoway and Booz Allen Hamilton, *Pan-Canadian Electronic Health Record: Quantitative and Qualitative Benefits*, March 2005.

CHAPTER 13

page 418 **"The Institute of Medicine in the United States"**: The Institute of Medicine, *To Err Is Human: Building Safer Health System*. Washington, D.C.: National Academies Press, 2000.

Acknowledgements

We would like to thank the following individuals and organizations for assisting us in our work:

Marsha Barnes, Ministry of Health and Long Term Care, Ontario

Estera Bekier, MD, FRCPC

Ann Decter

Robert Elgie, C.M., LL.D., MD, FRCSC
Founder and First Director of **Dalhousie University's Health Law Institute**
Former Chair of the **Patented Medicine Prices Review**

Jeremy Friedman, MB, ChB, FRCPC
Head, Division of Pediatric Medicine, **The Hospital for Sick Children**
Associate Professor, Department of Pediatrics, **University of Toronto**

Cristina Grosso Gage, B.Sc. MBA
Clinical Research Manager
Juravinski Cancer Centre

Marvin H. Gans MD, FRCPC
Associate Professor of Pediatrics
Director of Pediatric Postgraduate Education
University of Toronto and **The Hospital for Sick Children**

Michael Gordon, MD, MSC, FRCPC
Former Vice President, Medical Services
Head of Geriatric and Internal Medicine
Baycrest Geriatric Health Care System

Beth Grosso

Michael Helewa, MD, FRCSC, FSOGC, FACOG
Professor, Faculty of Medicine, **University of Manitoba**
Site Medical Director, Woman and Child Program, **St. Boniface General Hospital**
Past President, **Society for Gynecology and Obstetrics of Canada**

Alyson Hewitt, Former Executive Director and Staff
Safe Kids Canada

Fred Holmes, B.Math
Former Senior Director, ONV Center of Excellence
Emergis Inc.

Lynda Kirby RN, LCCE
Birth and Postpartum Doula

Reg Kusnierczyk, MD

Glenn Lott, CA, B.Math
Partner
Lott & Company Chartered Accountants

Anna Porter

Selena Qi
Lawrence Decter Investment Counsel Inc.

Shirlee Sharkey, RN
President & CEO
Saint Elizabeth Healthcare

Beverly Slopen
Beverly Slopen Literary Agency

Susan Sue-Chan
Ministry of Health and Long Term Care: Ontario

Wendy Thomas
Editor

Sandra Tooze
Penguin Group (Canada)

Toby Trompeter Kraman
Grosso McCarthy Inc.

Diane Turbide
Penguin Group (Canada)

Tina Warren
Former Vice President
Strategic Communications and Public Affairs
The Hospital for Sick Children

Zoe Whittall

Ruth Wilson, MD

Jennifer Zelmer, PhD
Former Vice President
Canadian Institute for Health Information

Special thanks are owed to our families for their support, especially Geneviève and Riel Roch-Decter; Steve, Giulia, Zack, Henry, and Teddy Paikin; and Michael McCarthy for relentlessly doing double duty at Grosso McCarthy Inc. while this book was being written.

Index